Forever

Fit and Flexible

Forever
Fit and Flexible

**Feeling Fabulous at
Fifty and Beyond**

Cheryl L. Ilov

Forever Fit and Flexible: Feeling Fabulous at Fifty and Beyond
Published by Willow Bay Publishing
Denver, CO

Library of Congress Control Number: 2016944214
Ilov, Cheryl L., Author
Forever Fit and Flexible: Feeling Fabulous at Fifty and Beyond
Cheryl L. Ilov

ISBN: 978-0-9976813-0-7

Healthy Living
Women's Health

Cover Photograph by Vanessa Plouffé

QUANTITY PURCHASES: Schools, companies, professional groups, clubs, and other organizations may qualify for special terms when ordering quantities of this title. Email info@cherylilov.com, for information.

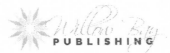

DEDICATION

This book is dedicated to the memory of Mr. Larry Boyette,
who was so much more than a ballet teacher and friend.
He taught me that there are no excuses, on the dance floor
or in life. Most of all, he was a gentleman,
and he taught me how to be a lady.
Anything less was simply unacceptable.

BALLET MASTER

The house lights grow dim
It's opening night
The audience quiets
Enter, stage right.

A spotlight appears
A bright, shining light
And follows the movement
Of one special life.

Of a ballet master
Mentor and friend
Artist, dancer
Elite gentleman.

His ageless elegance
Style and grace
A quiet reflection
Of a more gracious place.

Firm and determined
And true to his art
He follows these truths
With a compassionate heart.

These are the rules
There are no exceptions
There are no excuses
In this quest for perfection.

His students adore him
With respect, love, and fear
And they keep learning
With each passing year.

Of all of his students
Who have gone before
The last of his students
Could not love him more.

We continue to work
Each tendue, relevé
As we remember
His clean, precise way.

The curtains now close
We walk into the night
Our lives so much richer
Exit, stage right.

For Mr. Boyette, from a loving and grateful heart.
Cheryl Ilov, © March 2005

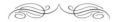

Contents

My Personal Journey to Fitness and Flexibility

I was fortunate enough to be relatively fit, flexible, and slender for most of my life. Or, at least I started out that way, and there was no reason to believe things would ever change. As a child, I never had to worry about my weight. I was so naturally slim and slight of build that it actually raised eyebrows when I was a kid.

Being of hearty Eastern European peasant stock, a solid build and sturdy constitution were very much admired as a sign of robust health and vitality. I fell far short of the ideal specimen in that department within my family. My paternal grandmother actually accused my mother of running out of food to provide me proper nourishment at the dinner table, since I was her third child in four years and the last one to get served. My mother jokingly told people that, even though I had a good appetite, I was so thin and delicate because I had a tapeworm living inside my body. I heard this so often that I believed it for a while and solemnly shared this bit of information with my kindergarten teacher on my first day of school. Good thing my teacher was a neighbor and knew my mother pretty well; otherwise, it could have been a real problem.

I was so much smaller than my two older sisters that they kept a close eye on me and often had to step in and protect me when the situation warranted. Since we were so close in age we often played together, and naturally I always tried to keep up with them. It got me into trouble on more than one occasion.

One instance happened during the summer I turned five. My parents were involved with getting the community swimming pool ready to open. The final step was to fill the pool from a huge water pipe. It was a brutally hot day, and my sisters and I were mesmerized by the swirling water as it gushed from the pipe and began to fill up the deep end of the pool. Since my parents and several other grownups were right there at the edge of the pool, they gave us permission to get in the water (fully clothed, of course) and cool off as the pool continued to fill. It seemed like a great idea to have the distinct honor of being the first ones in the pool before the season even opened.

Everything started out fine, until the water began to saturate my clothes and weigh me down. I struggled to stay afloat, but I got caught in the whirlpool. I started going under and frantically reached for the ledge around the deep end, but my fingers kept slipping off. Between the weight of my clothes, my small frame, the swirling water, and the slippery ledge, I was in serious trouble. My sisters were only slightly less hysterical than I and took turns pushing me up toward the ledge as they screamed to the adults for help. My dad jumped in and pulled me to safety, but it was my sisters who sounded the alarm and kept my head above water for those few desperate seconds.

Later that same summer, our family was at a church picnic, which happened to be at the local amusement park. All of us kids were in heaven as we ran from ride to ride. We finally came to the pride of the park, the roller coaster named "The Mad Mouse." It had individual cars instead of a chain of cars linked together like a train. The track included a series of bumps toward the end of the ride, each one a little bigger than the previous.

Since I was the smallest child, I was put in a car with my oldest sister, sitting in front of her with her legs wrapped around me and both of us holding onto the safety bar. It was great fun until we got to the series of bumps. I was so light that when we hit the first bump I flew up into the air between my sister and the safety bar and landed halfway out of the car. My sister grabbed me and tried to pull me back into the car as we hit the second bump. I flew even higher into the air and landed further out of the car, bent at the waistline, with my fingers dangling just a few inches from the track.

Even in my panic, I could feel my sister desperately grabbing at the only thing she could get ahold of—the waistband of my underpants. I could see all of the grownups screaming from below, including my mother, who was seven months pregnant. Bless her heart, she was running beside the tracks with her arms outstretched as if she'd be able to catch me. That's when I knew I was in a precarious situation. In my entire young life, I had never seen my mother run or try to catch anything. Fortunately, my sister's strength and the elastic of my underpants both held out as we hit the third bump. By that time, the young man operating the ride realized what was happening and slowed the ride down as it came into the station. The poor guy was white and shaking as he picked me up and handed me over to my parents. So was my sister. My mother didn't look so good, either. It might have been the pregnancy, but I suspect the possibility of losing her youngest child drained the blood right out of her face. Fortunately, my sister had quick reflexes and my new underwear had strong elastic, so my life was preserved. However, even now my sister can't talk about that day at the park without getting sick to her stomach.

The rest of the summer passed without further incident until it was time for me to start school. I walked to school with my two older sisters, but always walked home with my second oldest, since our older sister got out of school later than the two of us. I remember one particularly windy and blustery day when I needed to walk home by myself. My sister had a Brownie Scout meeting after school and had already asked permission for me to attend the meeting with her, so we could walk home together afterwards. She was informed that the meetings were for the troop members only, and I wouldn't be able to attend a meeting until I joined the Brownie Scouts the following year. *That's okay*, I thought to myself. It would be kind of nice to be on my own. After all, between my two older sisters and a new baby at home, I rarely got any time to myself. I was looking forward to flying solo, so to speak.

I had just started to head home, when my sister appeared out of nowhere, grabbed my hand, and informed me that she was taking me with her to her meeting. I asked her why and she replied, "It's too windy outside. I don't want you to blow away." She was serious! She pulled me into the meeting with her, stood me in front of her troop leader, and, in her most grownup voice, informed the woman that I *would* be attending the meeting after all, since the wind would surely blow me away if she wasn't there to hold me down.

To this day, I have a mental image of my sister walking me home and holding on to my hand as I flew behind her like a kite—with my skirt around my ears and my Mary Janes dancing in the wind. Yes, I was that skinny. As a matter of fact, my father's nickname for me was "Skinny," and I was too young to mind or care. In actuality, being skinny was kind of cute on a little girl that young, especially once my mother assured everyone that she was indeed feeding me, and no, I did not really have a tapeworm.

By the time I got to junior high school, being that thin was no longer cute. It was kind of embarrassing actually, especially when the other girls started to develop, if you know what I mean. My clothes swung on me like they were hanging on a hanger, while my classmates were beginning to fill theirs out in very interesting and provocative ways. My mother began a campaign to fatten me up, which included buying a box of Reese's peanut butter cups (my favorites) and putting them in the freezer for me to snack on. Not only did I have an entire box of frozen candy bars all to myself, my mom encouraged me to eat as many as I wanted, no questions asked. I guess she figured there was enough protein in the peanut butter to justify loading me up on sugar. But when I opened the freezer that first evening to get my snack I was faced with an empty box. Apparently, my father and my three sisters had gotten to the box before me. When I showed my mother the empty box, she just shook her head and said, "Kid, you're on your own." And so I was. She assured us both that I would fill out in time.

By the time I got to high school, I was still extraordinarily thin and underdeveloped, but luckily I finally got a good pair of legs. Thanks to my gene pool, combined with the benefit of countless majorette practices, downhill skiing, competitive swimming, and a good padded bra (except when I was swimming), I started to develop a nice figure as well as a *fit and flexible* physique. Unbeknownst to me, however, college was right around the corner, and waiting for me there was not only the wonder of higher education, but the insidious onset of the "freshmen fifteen."

It didn't take long for me to pack on the pounds from sitting in class all day and studying all night. I suppose the late night pizzas and keg parties on the weekends didn't help much either. I got absolutely no exercise and it was really beginning to show.

Things began to change in my sophomore year when my cousin literally dragged me to my first ballet class. She had been nagging me for months to take a class with her, but I adamantly refused to go. My only previous formal dance experience consisted of one year of tap and ballet from the local dance teacher when I was four years old. As a child, it had been fun. Besides, I loved the sound of those tap shoes banging against the floor. But now, as an adult, ballet didn't sound like fun at all. In fact, it sounded grueling, and I was quite certain I would hate it.

Finally, one Saturday morning, my cousin showed up at my dorm room armed with an extra leotard and a pair of tights, along with a look of sheer determination on her face. There was no way I was getting out of it, so I resigned myself to the inevitable. Besides, the dance studio was off campus and a walk to town was always a treat, even if it was going to dead-end in a ballet class.

Much to my surprise, I loved the class. From that moment on, I was hooked. I found myself starting my ballet training at an age when most dancers are packing up their pointe shoes and retiring their tutus. I loved the physical aspect of ballet, as well as the artistic expression. Several of my friends laughed at me for taking up ballet so "late in life," but once they saw the results, they stopped laughing. Twice a week for the next three years, I walked to and from the dance studio for an hour-and-a-half class. All that walking and dancing nicely balanced out the beer and pizza for the remainder of my college career.

I discovered Pilates after I graduated and moved to Denver. My ballet master highly recommended Pilates for all of his students to help them improve their dance technique as well as their strength and flexibility. I had no idea what Pilates was or why I would possibly want to do it, but I knew that if Mr. Boyette said to do something there was usually a good reason behind it. Besides, we were all so terrified of him back in those days that we would do almost anything he told us to do, as long as it wasn't illegal, immoral, or unethical.

Mr. Boyette had a reputation for being strict with his dancers, which was an understatement. He could bring a dancer to tears with just a look, let alone a verbal dressing down. It was rumored that he even had a mahogany stick that he used to poke the dancers with at the barre when they displeased him. Now, I never saw the stick, and I never really believed the story until years later when I heard him joking about it in a class with several of his longtime students. He casually remarked, "I wonder what happened to that stick?" One of the dancers replied, "It's hanging over my fireplace!" The entire room erupted in laughter. Maybe the stories were true after all, but I didn't want to take a chance, so I did what he said and enrolled in Pilates classes just in case.

After my move to Denver, I found myself in ballet class four days a week and in Pilates class two days a week. I was in my mid-twenties and back to my slender, fit, and flexible self. I figured I was set for life and would never have to worry about my weight or fitness the way other people did. Unfortunately, what I envisioned and what came to pass were two entirely different things. And when reality hit, it hit me hard. At the tender young age of thirty-five, I began to struggle with my weight, fitness, and flexibility.

My downhill spiral began with a slow, insidious onset of discomfort and tightness in my low back. I tried not to pay attention to it, thinking that if I ignored it, the discomfort would eventually go away on its own. I was wrong. The tightness gradually progressed to sharp pain that shot across my lower back, which I tried to alleviate with stretching and hot packs. That worked about as well as ignoring the problem. Before I knew it, I had pain radiating across my back, into my right buttock, searing into my hip joint, and burning down my leg.

Ironically, my back pain happened to coincide with my decision to go back to school to earn my master's degree in physical therapy. Since I had to complete a long list of required classes before I could even apply to graduate school, something had to give in my schedule. I gave up my Pilates workouts and drastically cut back my ballet classes from four times a week to two times a week. At least, I tried to go twice a week. There were weeks where I did nothing but work, study, and go to school. And that's when the trouble began.

Sitting is evil, and so is a sedentary lifestyle. My body

rebelled against the sudden inactivity, but I didn't realize it at the time. I was so focused on achieving my goal to get into physical therapy school, I couldn't think of anything else. When my pain got severe enough, however, I couldn't help but think about it then. It was always on my mind because I was in constant pain, day and night.

For two-and-a-half long and miserable years, I lived the nightmare of being a chronic pain patient. Not only did I have constant, incapacitating pain, I also had to bear the hopeless indignity of being told by multiple healthcare providers and experts in their field that I would never recover. I went to medical doctors, chiropractors, physical therapists, and massage therapists. Nothing worked. One well-meaning, but terribly misguided, expert told me that the arthritis in my spine was so severe I would never be able to do my grocery shopping and my laundry on the same day. She even suggested that I apply for disability. When I told her that my goal was to get back into ballet class, she actually snickered and said, "You're not eighteen anymore!" I wanted to slap her, but I was in too much pain.

Pain is a harsh but powerful teacher. If I had listened to the warning signs my body was sending me, I would have been able to interrupt the cycle of pain before it got so out of control.

It was a long, frustrating, and difficult road to recovery, but I did recover. Along the way I learned a lot about finding the path to health and healing. However, in the process my metabolism came to a screeching halt. I had gained weight and lost a tremendous amount of muscle strength and tone. My energy and stamina plummeted. Just the simple act of walking up a flight of stairs made my heart pound, my legs cramp, and left me wheezing like a freight train. Even though I was pain-free, my spine was stiff and inflexible, and my back muscles were incredibly tight. I wasn't able to bend forward, backward, or side to side. Not only had I lost all flexibility in my spine, but also in my legs, hips, and even my neck and shoulders. I couldn't believe what bad shape I was in, and I wondered how that could possibly have happened. I thought that once I recovered from my injury I would be right where I was before the injury occurred. I was wrong, and now I had to figure out what to do about it.

It was time to try and get my body back. I threw out the boring and tedious stretches and exercises that my physical therapists had given me, since they weren't helping me anyway. I started doing my Pilates mat exercises, being careful to move slowly and carefully, paying close attention to my movements, and listening to the messages my body was giving me as guidance. I pulled out a book I had on Pilates, reviewed the six basic principles of Pilates, and tried to implement those principles in every move I made. Instead of just doing the exercises I *embodied* them and spent just as much time on my mental conditioning as the physical aspect of Pilates. That was a lesson well learned from my past experiences and formal training, and, as a result, my change in tactics began to pay off.

My own body began to give me much better information and feedback than any of the experts I had worked with along the way. After a few months of doing my self-guided Pilates rehabilitation, I decided to give ballet class a try. I went back to class and stood in an obscure corner in the back of the room. Again, I moved slowly and thoughtfully, always stopping or modifying the movement pattern when I felt any discomfort. On my first day back I only made it through the first few barre exercises before my body gave me very clear signals that I had done enough. At least it was a start.

For the first three weeks, I could only get through the first twenty minutes of class before my body and my brain told me it was time to stop. In keeping with my newfound awareness and sensitivity, I listened to those inherent messages and left class. The dancers made sympathetic sounds my way as I left, and the looks of pity followed me out the door. What they didn't know was that I didn't need anyone's sympathy because I felt triumphant. I was twenty minutes further ahead than I had been three weeks earlier, and that was a huge accomplishment for me.

Eventually my twenty minutes expanded into thirty, and finally I could manage to successfully get through a forty-five minute barre. I began to regain some of the strength, fitness, and flexibility I had lost. However, before I was able to make any significant and permanent progress, I was accepted into the physical therapy master's program at Colorado University. It was a happy day, but it also meant that I would now be in school full-time, eight hours a day, five days a week, for two whole years to complete my master's degree. Just the thought of it was simultaneously thrilling and terrifying, but I looked at the bright side. I thought that becoming a physical therapist would be a terrific way to help people move better, feel better, and get out of pain, while I learned how to heal myself and get back into shape at the same time. It turned out I was only half right.

I found it fascinating that a program designed to teach sixty physically active individuals how to keep people healthy through exercise would immobilize these same people in a classroom for eight hours a day, five days a week. My exercises of choice had always been ballet and Pilates classes. Yet, driving across town from campus to ballet class or to the Pilates studio meant carving out three hours from my day that I simply could not afford to lose from my study time. Nor could I afford to pay for the classes even if I did find the time, having no income as a full-time graduate student.

Some of my classmates were runners, and I really envied them. They could grab their running shoes, lace them up, and enjoy a great thirty-minute run during lunch. Those who liked working out at a gym had a nice facility right there on campus, at no cost to them. A quick trip to the gym did wonders for their fitness and well-being. My classmates were kind enough to invite me to join them, but I was, and still am, allergic to running—and the thought of working out in a gym makes me break out in hives. Unless the university opened up a ballet school or Pilates studio, I was out of luck. So, instead of moving, I sat once again.

I turned sitting into a fine art. I sat in class, listened to lectures, and took notes during the day. I sat at home, transcribed my notes, and studied in the evening. I sat in the library for hours on end and studied during the weekend. I got a lot smarter from all that studying, but I also got stiffer, heavier, and more sluggish.

Even worse, my back began to give me very specific signals that it was not happy with all that sitting. As I said, pain is a powerful teacher, so this time I listened to the messages my body was sending me. To prevent myself from sliding back into the dark pit of chronic pain, I would get down on the floor of the lecture hall or on one of the treatment tables in the lab several times a day to do my gentle Pilates exercises. It was a source of great entertainment and amusement to my classmates, who referred to them as my "old lady exercises."

They changed their minds once I taught them some of the exercises and they discovered that the exercises were too hard for them to do. Score one for the old lady!

Other than that, the only exercise I ever got was walking to and from my car each day. The only strength training I got was lifting a heavy backpack filled with textbooks and enough comfort food to get me through a grueling and stressful fourteen-hour day. During midterms and finals I was able to enjoy a few brisk jaunts across the street to the local 7-11 for a quick junk food fix to satisfy even the most desperate graduate student.

Always the optimist, I tried not to worry about the lack of exercise, the weight gain, loss of flexibility, and occasional back spasms that threatened to spiral out of control if I wasn't careful. I figured I could get back into shape soon after graduation. After all, how difficult could it be? I graduated three months before my fortieth birthday and returned to ballet class with all the enthusiasm and naiveté of someone who did not have a clue what it meant to be forty and out of shape after four years of immobility.

My first class back to the ballet studio was a complete disaster and a harsh reality check. Not only had I gained even more weight during graduate school, I was shocked to see how much more flexibility I had lost. When I started graduate school, I had made considerable progress in my fitness and flexibility although I wasn't nearly where I had been before my back pain. But by the time I completed the program, I had lost what improvement I had gained, and more. Just wiggling into my leotard and tights was a workout in itself and an accident waiting to happen. And that was before class even started! After two years of sitting, my posture was horrible. I couldn't even stand up straight, no matter how hard I tried.

After two years of studying, I could remember all of my anatomy and physiology, but I couldn't remember basic, simple dance combinations. Even my balance, coordination, and reflexes had deteriorated while I was in physical therapy school, and I trudged along like I was moving through wet cement.

Obviously, I forgot about the awareness and sensitivity I had learned when I recovered from my back injury, because I doubled my efforts and vowed to work harder. I was rewarded with muscle spasms, hip pain, and a torn calf muscle. I even tore my triceps doing grand battement (big leg kicks) while standing at the barre. It's not unusual for a dancer to strain or pull a leg muscle doing grand battement if they are not properly warmed up, since it's the leg muscles that do all the heavy lifting, so to speak. But it is absolutely unheard of to tear an arm muscle! The hand is merely resting gently on the barre, or is supposed to be, rather than hanging on for dear life the way I was the day I tore my triceps.

I was so out of shape that I couldn't properly stand on my left leg, so I compensated with a white-knuckled grip on the barre with my left hand. When I kicked my right leg up, my body lurched backward. To correct myself, I abruptly yanked myself upright with my left arm. I immediately felt a sharp pain and strange spasm in my left upper arm, causing me to drop to the floor like a stone. Apparently I had over-corrected. There was a stunned silence as the dancers watched me writhe on the floor in pain, clutching my left arm with my right hand. Eventually one of my barre buddies recovered her composure enough to ask me if I was okay. "No," I replied through clenched teeth, "I think I tore my triceps." Our teacher rolled her eyes, gave me a look that was a combination of disbelief and disgust and bellowed, "Other side!" Over the years I have discovered that some dance teachers have no empathy.

I hauled myself up to a standing position with my good arm, careful not to jerk too hard on the barre. I continued the class with my left arm dangling helplessly at my side until I couldn't stand the pain any longer. Two days later, I had a multi-colored bruise from my armpit to my elbow. This was a ballet injury that would go down in history, and I was the talk of the town among the ballet community for weeks. As a result of that injury, I was reminded of an important lesson I had already learned from my Pilates training as well as my physical therapy training—lurching movements damage muscles and joints. Smooth, flowing movements are much more conducive to healthy movement. It was a powerful lesson to remember, but I wish it had been a little less painful and a lot less embarrassing.

In retrospect, I realize I had gone back to my old ways of approaching every obstacle put in my way ... by forcing my way through them. I'm not sure if I forgot everything I taught myself after my back injury, or if physical therapy school scrambled my brain so much that I couldn't think straight. Either way, instead of listening to my body and the signals it was giving me, I ignored them just like I had done when I experienced the early signs of a devastating back injury. This time my body was even less forgiving about my mistakes than it had been a few years earlier.

Obviously, I was a train wreck and I needed serious help. What was even more frustrating was that as a dancer and a physical therapist, I could not figure this out on my own, and I didn't even know why. Everything that had worked for me regarding fitness when I was in my twenties and thirties was simply not working now. It was like all of the rules had suddenly been changed overnight and nobody thought to mention them to me. I was faced with a serious challenge, but at

least I was fortunate enough to be working in the ideal pro-
fession, where help was right at my fingertips and just a few
steps away. I was surrounded by coworkers who were ready,
willing, and able to help me. Or so I thought.

My first job as a physical therapist was at a busy rehabilitation
hospital. A young male colleague heard me moaning about
my struggles to lose weight and get back into some sort of
shape. He just happened to be a personal trainer as well as
a physical therapist and had plenty of experience and success whipping people back into shape. He offered to take
me on as his personal project. He designed a weight training
program for me, using free weights that I could do at home. I
went along with him and his plan, realizing that I had nothing
to lose but some extra pounds. I did think that the amount of
weight he wanted me to lift was too heavy, especially considering the torn triceps that had resulted from just holding on
to the ballet barre. Still, I was willing to give it a try, because
he did seem to know what he was talking about. He did have
all of that experience as a personal trainer, so I figured he
must know *something* that I didn't know.

He lost me, though, when he told me that I simply had to
eat more to lose weight. I lost him when I laughed in his face
and asked him if he had ever been a woman over forty. In
reality, I wasn't laughing at him; I was laughing at myself. To
this day, I am quite certain he knew what he was doing and
that he had all of the best intentions. However, my natural
sass and smarty pants came out when I realized that he had
never been a woman over forty, nor had he ever worked with
one. His experience as a trainer was with young men who
wanted to buff up, not middle-aged ladies who were horribly

out of shape. For these reasons, I realized he probably was not the best person to help me. I tried to keep my sense of humor, but it eventually became apparent that he didn't find my situation as amusing as I did. We recognized that we had very different philosophies as well as biologies, so we parted ways, once again leaving me to fend for myself.

Soon after that fiasco, a close friend of mine explained that I just needed to understand how my body and my metabolism were changing, and there simply was nothing I could do about it. A very smart lady, she always enjoyed educating me on the facts of life whenever the opportunity presented itself. She informed me that she had learned to accept the fact that some women she knew were now two sizes larger than they had been when they were younger. She recommended that I accept it as well. "After all, it does happen to almost everyone," she said with great authority.

To make matters worse, she reminded me that menopause was rapidly approaching and my metabolism was going to slow down even more. Terrific. In an attempt to cheer me up, she told me that we could walk down that road together. After all, misery loves company! She reasoned that if we just gave in, we could eat anything we wanted and not worry about it. For some reason, that did not lift my spirits.

I confided in a former classmate, explaining my dilemma and expressing my frustration. She listened patiently and made appropriate sympathetic clucking sounds as I bared my soul to her. When I finished, she smugly reminded me that I did, after all, have a forty-year-old body. What did I expect? I wanted to slap her across her twenty-six-year-old face. Instead, I restrained myself and tried to take comfort in the knowledge that she also would be forty someday. When I did the math, I realized I would be fifty-four at that time. And, considering the downhill slide I was on, it was not going to be pretty.

That is what finally did it: the cumulative effect of these three widely different viewpoints collided head-on with my own personal belief system and motivated me to take charge of my own destiny and follow my own instincts. I refused to go down without a fight, and my incomparable stubbornness kicked into high gear.

I stopped listening to everyone else and started listening to myself and my body instead. Rather than judging my body and how it looked, I changed my focus from how I wanted to *look* to how I wanted to *feel*. I adjusted my goal from trying to lose weight to no longer gaining weight. It was not a very lofty goal, but it was one that I thought I could accomplish. I tried a lot of different dietary changes and a variety of exercise techniques. I kept the things that felt right and ditched the ones that did not. In a relatively short timeframe, I had more energy, felt stronger, and had lost three pounds. Three pounds didn't seem like much, but I was encouraged. At least I now had hope.

My ballet master noticed the missing three pounds, and so did my doctor. They were both delighted. That encouragement was all I needed to light a fire under me. I felt I was finally on the right path and I continued my quest from there. I kept to my own personal truth of listening to myself while I educated myself on nutrition, a topic I had never really taken the time to learn about. I made a habit out of reading labels when I went to the grocery store, and began preparing healthier meals. I even kept a diary to help me stay on top of my game. I made a point to start moving and stay moving. When I was at work, I would get down on the floor and do a few exercises between clients. I got rid of my chair and replaced it with an exercise ball. When I did sit in a chair, I would do a few chair push-ups to strengthen and tone the muscles of my arms, especially the one I tore at the ballet barre. I moved slowly when I climbed up (and down) a flight of stairs to help strengthen and shape my legs. When I was cooking or cleaning the kitchen, I put on some music and boogied a bit as I did my household chores. I parked as far away from storefronts as possible every time I went shopping, as long as it was daylight. (No reason to take unnecessary risks). Don't misunderstand; I wasn't exercising every waking moment, but I discovered that just adding a few minutes of movement activities during the day made a huge difference in improving my weight, fitness, and flexibility.

As time passed, I did encounter additional physical challenges. Since my episode of low back pain and consequent recovery, I was diagnosed with three additional chronic pain syndromes over the years. Each time was as much of a living hell as the previous one, and each time I was told that I would have to learn how to live with the pain. I was told I would have to alter my lifestyle to accommodate the pain and side effects of the medications. I would also need to allow time in my schedule for the many necessary doctor's appointments and treatments. But, every time, I managed to claw my way back to a full recovery.

In every case, the problem was caused by a musculo-skeletal imbalance rather than some disease process. I recovered with the aid of alternative therapies, including acupuncture and naturopathic medicine. However, the most powerful healing process came from correcting faulty movement patterns that caused unnecessary stress and strain on my joints and muscles. It's hard to imagine what my life would be like if I had accepted the predictions of the "experts" who treated me.

I understand what it's like to wake up every morning and wonder if I'll ever be healthy and functional again. I know what it's like to be in incapacitating pain. I even know the indignity of being told that I am supposed to be overweight and have pain because it is a "natural" consequence of menopause and part of the "aging process." I can still feel the frustration of being told I would no longer be able to do the activities I loved because I was too injured and decrepit.

My life experiences and my body's wisdom taught me something different, however. It is possible to heal from anything, and there is an incredible healing power in movement. I discovered the art of healing through movement as I transformed myself into a *movement artist* rather than a physical therapist. I realized that exercise just for the sake of exercise isn't enough, especially for a population that is fifty and older. Of the many blessings that came out of my own awful experiences was a path to health and healing that led me to discover two more remarkable movement arts: The Feldenkrais Method® and martial arts. Everything I've lived through led me to integrate the principles of Pilates, Feldenkrais®, dance, and martial arts to create a program that brought me back to a life of health, vitality, fitness, flexibility, and an ideal weight. At the age of fifty-nine, I love the way I look, move, and feel. My personal journey to fitness and flexibility has been long and arduous, but incredibly enlightening and rewarding at the same time. It led me to know firsthand that it is possible to thrive and feel vibrantly alive at fifty and beyond and to bring together a set of powerful tools to create a program that can benefit others.

Your Journey to Becoming
Forever Fit and Flexible

Imagine waking up every morning with a spring in your step and an eager anticipation of the day ahead. Consider what it would be like to get out of bed and be able to move with ease and elegance as you glide around your kitchen to prepare for your day. Picture yourself stepping out of the shower and liking what you see in the full-length mirror before you get dressed. Now visualize that you can engage in any activity you want to do (and love to do) with strength, grace, and confidence. Think of what it would be like to hike without hip pain, golf without back pain, dance without knee pain, or get down on the floor (and back up again) to play with your grandkids. Imagine a new sense of energy and vitality that

you never thought possible as you move into your fifties, sixties, seventies, and beyond. Yes, this could be your future,
and yes, it *is* possible. As a matter of fact, the possibilities are
endless, and you have already taken the first step by opening
the pages of *Forever Fit and Flexible.* As you move through
the sections and chapters ahead, here is a glimpse of what
you'll discover.

Part One introduces the foundations of the *Forever Fit
and Flexible* program. In Chapters One through Three, we
address the power of using your attention and awareness to
help you achieve your goals and accomplish the maximum
benefit from the movement lessons included in later chapters. We also discuss the impact of positive thinking, including having the right mindset and surrounding yourself with
positive people. Along those same lines, never underestimate the power of your imagination and visualization. After
all, what we believe is what we become.

Several years ago my husband and I were traveling to At-
lanta to visit his family. We were on the train from the con-
course to baggage claim, and I was practicing a technique I
learned in martial arts. I stood with my knees bent, my eyes
closed, and without holding on to anything, I practiced finding my balance while I sensed the movement of the train. As
I was getting into a meditative state, I heard a loud voice say,
"I have to sit down because I'm an old lady! When you're an
old lady, you can sit down, too." I opened my eyes and saw a
woman squeezing into the last available seat and talking to a
little girl standing near her. I closed my eyes again and went
back to my musings and practice while the woman continued
her litany about being an old lady. When we got off the train
and moved toward the escalators, I automatically went to the
stairs while the woman continued, "I have to take the escala-

tor because I'm an old lady!" *Good grief,* I wondered, *How old is this lady, anyway?* I turned around to look at her and almost fell the rest of the way down the stairs. The woman had to be at least ten years younger than I was at the time! What kind of message was she sending to herself, not to mention the little girl, who was clinging to her mother's hand and staring at this woman with eyes as huge as saucers? Getting older is inevitable—being old is a choice. With *Forever Fit and Flexible,* you have the opportunity to grow older gracefully without becoming *old.*

In Chapter Four, we focus in depth on the principles of each of the four movement arts—Pilates, Feldenkrais, dance, and martial arts—including the powerful health and fitness benefits of each method. I share the foundations of each method and weave them into the movement lessons presented. I invite you to take your time as you go through each chapter and work with each method and the various techniques. Some of these movement lessons will work for you, and some of them will not.

Chapter Five outlines the eight fundamental principles of the *Forever Fit and Flexible* program for you to follow. There are also strategies for how to work through the movement lessons to best accommodate your learning style.

Incorporating the principles of Pilates, Feldenkrais, dance, and martial arts, I have developed the system *Forever Fit and Flexible* and designed a variety of movement lessons for you to do at home. Each movement lesson in the program is founded in one of these remarkable movement arts.

The chapters presented in Part Two address the individual components that are essential to your journey to fitness and flexibility. Each chapter provides specific movement lessons related to that component, such as posture, core strength, flexibility, balance, and strengthening. You will learn why each is important and the role each plays in your process.

Once you have established a solid foundation by following the building blocks in Chapters Six through Nine, we progress to the next steps by adding the bricks and mortar to your structure, which include functional strengthening and movement. I use the term "functional strengthening," because you will learn how to use basic functional activities that you can engage in multiple times a day to incorporate into your *Forever Fit and Flexible* program.

After you have developed your posture, core strength, flexibility, balance, and functional strengthening, we will look at the many opportunities you have to start moving and stay moving. You can engage in a variety of different activities that you actually enjoy, so that it feels like you are playing and having fun rather than digging ditches. When you participate in activities that you enjoy, you are far more likely to keep up with them.

The final part of building a *Fit and Flexible* program is the area of nutrition. You can't have a strong, healthy body if you don't provide the proper fuel to keep it running smoothly. There are plenty of gimmicks advertised that are easy to fall prey to, just like my clients who were replenishing their workouts with high calorie and sugar-loaded "health" drinks and "fit" bars. Beginning from this point forward, I encourage you to put the emphasis on self-education. Start reading labels very carefully when you go to the grocery store or try a new product such as protein bars or other "healthy" snacks. Our focus within the *Fit and Flexible* program will be on nutrition, not diets. Just hearing the word makes me shudder and conjures up the memory of my client's weight loss group. Going on a diet is not a recipe for success, but having a good understanding of healthy nutrition will lead you to success. It is also much better for your health.

As you go through this process, I encourage you to keep a journal and take notes to help you track your progress. Not only will this practice slow you down, it will help you integrate the mind-body connection that the *Forever Fit and Flexible* program is based upon. When you write down your observations and experiences, your brain has the opportunity to take in and process the information. Your brain then activates the motor and sensory pathways associated with your experiences and accelerates your progress.

I learned about the benefits of recording what happens, and my responses, reactions, and "take-aways" from what I learned, during my martial arts training; however, I didn't realize what a powerful tool this was until later in my training. As a matter of fact, in the beginning, when I first got on the mat, I wasn't even sure how to keep a journal or why I would possibly want to. When I began my training, I honestly thought I was embarking on a new form of recreation—until I discovered how serious these people were about their training. I mean, they had *notebooks*, for heaven's sake!

I wondered why they needed notebooks until I was given a few sheets of paper that listed the techniques I was responsible to learn before I tested for my yellow belt. I still didn't connect the dots, but I put the papers in a thin binder so as not to look out of place or to appear disrespectful. I brought the binder with me to each class, but I never made a single note inside, because I didn't have a clue about what I should write down or why—not even when I took my first three-day martial arts seminar.

My teacher brought his Sensei[1] out from L.A. to help us train. He had previously talked me into attending the seminar, even though I was only a yellow belt. He assured me that it would be fun and that Sensei was just like a great big teddy bear. Unfortunately, on the first day of the seminar, the great big teddy bear yelled and screamed at us all day about everything. Just when I thought he had surely run out of things to yell about, he bellowed at us for not taking notes. All of the upper belts whipped out their notebooks and began frantically writing. I pulled out a piece of paper and a pen and stared down at the sheet of paper. My mind was as blank and empty as the paper. I had no idea what I was supposed to write about. I tried to sneak a peek at the notes of the brown belt sitting next to me, but as far as I was concerned, he could have been writing in Japanese. Then I realized that he was. I was at a complete and utter loss.

I was ready to throw in the towel and put my notes aside until I noticed the great big teddy bear scowling at me. That wasn't a good sign, so I picked up my pen and paper and nervously began to write "bread, eggs, milk." After all, I didn't want to be the only one staring off into space, especially after *that* lecture. I figured no one would notice that I started my grocery list, because my handwriting is so bad that I was certain no one could possibly read it. I looked up from my list, thinking enough time had passed, but everyone was still scribbling notes, so I started planning my menu for the following week. Since I was already working on my grocery list, it was a natural segue. Finally, the notetaking period was over and we started practicing our techniques again. Every now and then, one of the guys would step off the mat, pick up his

1. In martial arts, Sensei is the word for teacher.

notebook, and jot down a few more notes. Not wanting to be outdone, I walked over to my notebook and wrote down a few more items that I needed from the grocery store.

That was twelve years ago, and since that time I have learned to record my thoughts and personal experiences in a variety of different classes and activities. I keep a small notebook in my purse, because I never know when I will have an *aha! moment* or inspiring idea. I keep my notebook beside me in ballet class, because the practice of making notes greatly improved my dance technique, and I can't help but wonder how many injuries I might have avoided if I had kept a journal all along. As a result, I now have copious notes that I can refer to whenever I get stuck or need to review a technique or a concept. I have also discovered the value of putting things down in writing. It certainly gives a person a lot to think about.

As you learn and practice these new techniques, check in with your mental and physical responses and record them. Never underestimate the power of the written word, especially when you put them down in your own voice. If you're not sure what to write down, start with your grocery list and go from there. Believe me, you'll figure it out.

Take time for mindful reflection and record those thoughts as well. Evaluate where you have been prior to beginning the program, where you are at the present moment, your progress and your experiences with the movement lessons, and how they are working for you. Identify and continue to work with the movement lessons that work for you and toss out the ones that do not. I encourage you to experiment with designing a program of your own that is customized to you, your body, and your needs. No matter what you modify, however, remember to stay true to the basic principles you learn within the *Fit and Flexible* program, because they are what make this so effective.

Along with keeping a journal, I suggest that you record the movement lessons in your own words and your own voice. First, read the directions and try the movement lessons a few times until you begin to get a feel for them and discover the points that are most relevant to you, including areas that you want to emphasize. Then, record the lesson. In this way, when you play back the recording, you will be able to focus more completely on your movements and your sensations as you do the lesson, instead of trying to simultaneously read the instructions. It's another way you can light up your nervous system and be more attentive to what you are doing, as well as make the lesson your own. The *Forever Fit and Flexible* program is a blueprint for you to use "as is" as well as to expand the concepts and ideas to make them your own.

There is a lot of confusing and misleading information in the marketplace today regarding health and fitness, especially for people over fifty. Yet I know from personal experience and from working with others that as we age we can continue to enjoy a healthy, active, and vibrant lifestyle. We just have to be a lot smarter about how we go about it by paying attention to what we're doing and by listening to our bodies. It is the difference between exercising with brute force versus moving with finesse and an artistic quality. I often tell my clients that it is like comparing a work boot to a ballet slipper. A work boot is functional and definitely has its purpose, but a ballet slipper commands a level of delicate skill and sophistication, which requires you to work smarter, not harder.

As a result of working with the *Forever Fit and Flexible*

program, you will get stronger and more limber and move with an ease and grace that seems effortless. You will discover the artistic quality of movement rather than mindlessly pushing through movement patterns that can injure your muscles and destroy your joints. My goal is to help you avoid some of the most common traps and pitfalls along the way as you also learn how to become a movement artist and pay close attention to your movements and listen to your body. I also want to spare you some of the expense, frustrations, and disappointments that I experienced in my own journey.

I invite you now to turn the page and begin your personal discovery of the knowing that it is possible to be fit, flexible, and fabulous well into your fifties, sixties, seventies, and beyond. Believe it or not, it is easier than you may think, and it can be a lot of fun as well. Everything you'll discover within these pages will guide you to find your own way to be *Forever Fit and Flexible*. That is my hope and prayer for you.

PART ONE

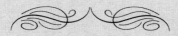

The Foundation

chapter one

Awareness is Your
Key to Success

"If you don't mind, it won't matter."

Before we dive into the methodology, techniques, and movement lessons of this program, there are some foundational concepts to consider. In the next five chapters, we will take a look at each one separately.

Near the end of the introduction, I referred to "movement lessons" rather than "exercises." That's because you are not just doing exercises; you will be *learning* new ways to move by fully engaging your mind and your body as you move. There are many reasons why the techniques in the *Forever Fit and Flexible* program are so powerful and effective, but the single most important component is very simple. It is *awareness*. Awareness is the capacity to pay attention—to focus your mind on yourself and your actions. It is a more alert state of consciousness, which increases your ability to understand your external surroundings and your internal feelings as well as your reactions to certain situations. It is a condition of being mindful.

Many traditional forms of exercise work your body but do not engage your mind. Mindless exercise definitely has its place. Walking on a treadmill, riding a stationary bike, or lifting weights will burn some calories. Likewise, they will increase your strength, build endurance, and generally improve your health to a certain degree. But mindless exercise will not give you the sleek, fit, flexible physique you are probably hoping for, a point that is illustrated through one of my clients.

When I met her, Jenna had been struggling with chronic low back pain and instability in her spine, something I could totally relate to. Once we began working together doing Pilates, her back pain completely resolved and her spine became stabilized. As an added bonus, her posture and her core strength dramatically improved. She even looked longer and leaner, and her clothes fit better. She became such a devoted follower of Pilates that she bought her own Pilates exercise equipment (the reformer) to use at home. She got on her reformer for a few minutes almost every day, and she looked and felt fabulous. She didn't need my help any longer, so we said our farewells.

A few years later, Jenna showed up at my office, complaining that she was gaining weight and getting thick around the middle. On top of that, her back pain was returning. She wailed that everything started going to hell in a handbasket after she hit the big Five-O. I cannot begin to tell you how many times I hear that exact same statement from new clients, both women and men alike.

Jenna also told me she was working so hard to get into shape that she had been taking a spin class three times a week for the past several months. Instead of losing weight and toning up, however, she was getting a flabbier stomach and thicker waistline, and was actually gaining more weight. That didn't sound right. I asked her if she was still using her reformer. She said she wasn't. The reformer had been relegated to an obscure corner of her basement. She had stopped using it because her back felt so good. Even though she had always enjoyed Pilates and felt great when she practiced it, she had gotten out of the habit of doing it. I asked her if she enjoyed her spin class. "No," Jenna replied, "I hate every minute of it!" I asked, "Then why are you doing it?" She responded, "Because it's supposed to be great exercise." I asked her how it was working out for her so far. She admitted that it wasn't.

It was time for her to change tactics. We got her back on her Pilates reformer and a daily walking program, which she enjoyed a whole lot more than going to spin class at the gym. After a few short weeks, Jenna once again appeared taller, leaner, and stronger. Her back pain disappeared and her joints felt more flexible, her tummy was flatter, and she was a lot happier. She even lost a little weight, which is really interesting since Pilates is not known for burning calories. I decided it was from the walking program, until I learned that the spin teacher encouraged her students to replenish themselves after class. She recommended that they use the protein bars and electrolyte drinks that the club sold, since they were losing so many vital nutrients during their workout. The instructor neglected to mention that the sugar and calorie content was so high that they were actually adding more calories than they burned. Rather than the spin-replenish regimen, they would have been better off sitting on the couch with a good book. Once Jenna eliminated the extra calories from her diet three days a week, she began to lose weight. I thought of my young colleague who wanted me to lift weights that were too heavy for me and insisted that I simply had to eat more to lose weight all those years ago. Obviously, there was a major disconnect between the enthusiastic young trainers and the fitness requirements of a population hitting fifty.

Over the next few months, I had two new clients who complained that they were getting soft and thick in the middle as well as experiencing back, hip, neck, and shoulder pain. Both of them were in their fifties and were taking a spin class three times a week, just like Jenna had done. And they apparently were getting the same results. They hated spin class just as much as she had but thought they should do it because it was supposed to be good for them. I honestly had to admire their dedication and persistence. I'm sure I would have thrown in the towel and headed for the closest doughnut shop after the first class. On the other hand, these ladies gave me a few things to think about. Maybe spin class wasn't the ideal exercise program for people in their fifties, especially if they hated it.

Cycling is fantastic exercise, but it puts us in a position of a rounded spine, or flexed posture. Not only does this put pressure on our spine, it pushes our abdominal muscles and soft tissues *out* rather than *in* and does not focus on strengthening our core muscles. Bicycling can also tighten our hips and bulk up our thighs. That's usually not the look that most of us are hoping for. If you do love to bike, you need to balance it out with activities that elongate and extend your spine, target your core muscles, and loosen your hip joints. We'll get into that in more detail in later chapters.

The movement lessons I have included in the *Forever Fit and Flexible* program aren't supposed to be done mindlessly, but with thoughtful attention to achieve the maximum benefit and a strong, flexible physique. You will get much more dramatic and longer-lasting results when you fully engage your brain during your physical activities, because you are training your mind and your awareness as well as your body. This awareness also transfers into other areas of your life to help you achieve your goals, make better decisions in your life and relationships, and simply get more pleasure and enjoyment out of life.

What I am referring to is called the mind-body connection, or what I like to call "mindful movements." Doing just fifteen minutes of the movement lessons in this book with thoughtful intention will benefit you more than one hour of mindless exercise at the gym. No matter how tempted you are to get through all of the exercises in the book, please stop yourself. I cannot emphasize enough how important it is to slow yourself down and really take your time with each chapter. Your body and your brain need time to integrate the movement patterns and the changes that you will experience. Yes, I said your brain. When you move with mindful awareness, you are actually training your brain to allow for these wonderful new changes to take place in your body. When you truly embody the mind-body connection, something magical begins to happen. You will achieve results much more quickly.

Each chapter in this book builds upon the previous one, and it is like putting together the pieces of a puzzle. Once you feel like you understand the basic principle of the chapter and the movement patterns that unfold as a result of practicing the movements presented, the lessons will begin to feel more natural, and you can then move on to the next chapter.

I suggest that you recruit a friend or two to go through this program with you if possible. By doing so, you can help and encourage each other and also share your progress. You can also support each other in discovering how best to tailor this program to your individual needs. Allow me to gently remind you to take notes and/or journal as you go through the chapters and experience the movement lessons. This really is a valuable practice to help you along the way. You may even want to put little reminders around your house, office, or workstation to help you move forward in mindful movement. Most of all, periodically remind yourself that you are *not* engaging in traditional exercise. You are practicing mindful movement—for life!

Awareness is your key to success in your *Forever Fit and Flexible* program. You are developing a life skill, and the more you practice it, the sharper it will become—in all aspects of your life. Just imagine what you can accomplish in each and every area of your life. The possibilities are endless, and awareness is the key!

chapter two

Mindset

"Attitude is everything."

Peter Pan had a point when he taught Wendy, John, and Michael how to fly. To reach their goal of taking flight, they had to think lovely thoughts. Without the right mindset, they were grounded. However, once they reached the right mental attitude, the sky was the limit, so to speak.

What we believe is what we become, and what we tell ourselves is what we believe. So, be careful what you tell yourself, and do not belittle yourself, even in jest. Negative, deprecating self-talk can do more harm to your self-image than you think and can quickly sabotage your efforts to get *fit and flexible*. I'm not talking about self-esteem; that is a completely different subject. Self-esteem refers to your sense of value and worth. Self-image, on the other hand, is how you see yourself from both an outward physical perspective and an internal one as well. The two are very closely related, and one does influence the other.

When I was a young girl, I was never very good at math, which I was reminded of repeatedly over the years by my teachers and my parents. I was also told that girls in general can't do math, and I certainly believed what I heard, because I had the grades to prove it. I began to believe that I wasn't necessarily stupid, but I definitely wasn't very smart, especially when it came to mathematics. As a result, I began to act dumb in class, especially when I didn't understand the material, which was most of the time.

In high school, I was fortunate enough to have a kind and patient algebra teacher who was able to explain the basic principles of algebra. As a result of that help, I passed his class with flying colors. However, that internal perception of being a mathematical moron stayed with me and came roaring back when I decided to pursue my master's degree in physical therapy. When I discovered that I had to take several college physics courses, I had a full-blown panic attack. I couldn't even do basic arithmetic, let alone the complicated equations waiting to derail me in a college physics class! The old but familiar internal story that I was stupid kept repeating itself in my mind. I reinforced this self-dialogue with my behavior, which was to act dumb and go into full avoidance mode, giving up my goal of becoming a physical therapist.

I looked into several other advanced degrees, but each one required the same physics courses. Damn! After weeks of agonizing over what to do, I came up with a plan. I could take the most simple, basic introductory college algebra class at the local community college. If I struggled, I could hire a tutor and join a study group. If I failed miserably, I would ditch my plans for graduate school. If I passed the class, I would advance to the major league at the university and take the regular college algebra course.

Not only did I ultimately pass, but I was able to help my classmates who were struggling with the material. I got the highest grade in the class, as I did in every math class after that, including algebra, trigonometry, statistics, and intro to calculus. I took intro to calculus just for fun, because I could. I discovered that not only was I good in math after all, but I absolutely loved it!

Here is another and more dangerous example is how our self-image can become distorted by the messages we receive. Over the years, I have seen several young, healthy, and promising young dancers succumb to the terrible disease of anorexia and bulimia. There can be a variety of situations that trigger an eating disorder, but an impressionable young girl trying to achieve the "ideal" body of a ballet dancer is most definitely one of the more powerful ones.

An off-hand comment made by a teacher, a parent, or even another dancer can start the downhill spiral. The positive attention the dancer receives from losing a few pounds reinforces the behavior and the belief that if she is thin, she is good; if she is heavy, she is bad. If she loses more weight, she's even better. A dangerous and frightening cycle has begun, and if it isn't interrupted immediately, she can suffer with the eating disorder for the rest of her (or his) life. This becomes part of her self-image, in the same way that part of mine was to believe I was stupid. I can offer a lot more examples, but I'm sure by now you are already coming up with some of your own. The sabotage of our self-image can occur in many different ways, and oftentimes, happens as a result of subtle circumstances.

Much of our self-image is deeply embedded in our belief system. It can be influenced by the messages we've received from society and our friends, and what we tell ourselves *about* ourselves. Self-image can even be as a result of what the experts, who may be trying to help us, tell us. What we tell ourselves is what we believe, and what we believe is what we become. Perhaps this is one of the reasons I managed to fight so hard to recover from my chronic pain syndromes. Deep down in my core belief system, I could not see myself as a chronic pain patient, no matter how many "experts" tried to convince me otherwise.

It's important, therefore, to be mindful of the company you keep. Negative people can weigh you down and even undermine your efforts to be physically, mentally, and emotionally healthy. Remember my friend who tried to convince me that we could walk down menopause lane together and not worry about how we looked or what we ate? Once I adopted a more positive attitude, started to lose weight and get in shape, our friendship quickly deteriorated. It's unfortunate, and for a long time I couldn't figure out why our relationship ended. Then I realized that as my body was getting stronger, so were my mind and strength of character. I wasn't in quite the same headspace that I had been in when we were friends, and we were no longer compatible.

Surround yourself with people who are positive and upbeat. Change the way you look at yourself, talk to yourself, and think about yourself. Learn and practice the art of self-compassion. It is so much better for your overall health and well-being. Consider the alternative and the damage you do when you do not treat yourself with kindness and gentle understanding. The following story is a fascinating example of what I'm talking about.

Several years ago, one of my clients invited me to speak to her weight loss group. Helen absolutely loved the group, even though she didn't have much success with losing weight. She felt like it was a wonderful support group and that it promoted positive reinforcement to make good choices. When I arrived at the meeting, the members all greeted me enthusiastically. The energy in the room was electric and I thought, *Wow, what a great group of people!* To start the meeting, the members stood up to recite a pledge, which they did before every meeting, right from their "members only" handbook. I thought it was a nice way to kick off their meeting, establish a sense of community, and focus on their goals. Besides, I thought it was kind of cute, just like the Girl Scout Creed we learned from our handbooks and recited at the beginning of our meetings all those years ago.

However, I was horrified once they began to speak and I heard their words. I don't remember the specific details, but included in the pledge were references to their being lazy, disgusting, and slothful. There was also a statement expressing that everyone they met would see their shame and lack of willpower because of their weight. *Yikes!* I listened in jaw-dropping disbelief as this beautiful group of people verbally abused themselves. The most powerful memory for me was how the energy in the room began to change, and how everyone seemed to wither, shrink, and go inward as they recited their pledge.

After the meeting, I suggested that perhaps they could change the wording of their pledge to include more positive and uplifting messages. My suggestion was not well-received, and I was never invited back to speak to the group. It is interesting to note that Helen never did lose weight when she was with that group. Apparently, neither did anyone else, and within a few months, the group disbanded. Helen continued to work with me, but she missed her group and still wanted to lose weight. Eventually she settled on Weight Watchers, and after a few months she was on her way to her ideal weight. I often wonder what the members of her other group could have accomplished if they had simply treated themselves with more respect.

I must confess that I used to engage in negative, deprecating self-talk myself. I was pretty good at it. As a matter of fact, I was a master at it and took it to a high art form. However, this self-sabotaging practice began to change once I began my Feldenkrais training. Feldenkrais has a way of peeling away the layers of self-doubt and untruths about ourselves that we acquire along the way over the years. Some people compare this process to peeling an onion. I disagree with that analogy, because when you peel an onion you never quite get to the end, and every layer makes you cry. Instead, I prefer to think of this process as peeling an artichoke. The protective outer layers that develop as an artichoke matures are thick, course, and prickly. However, once you peel back the outer layers, each layer underneath gradually becomes softer, more pliable, and more tender. Finally, you get to the best part of the artichoke, the heart. That's what Feldenkrais does for you—it brings you back to your true self and teaches you the art, and the heart, of self-respect and self-compassion.

As a result of this gentle process of unfolding, on my journey to becoming a Feldenkrais practitioner, I felt happier, healthier, and more energetic. I even felt younger, because the method also has a way of liberating your playful, childhood spirit and makes everything in life more fun again. I even discovered that I liked myself more, and I became my own best friend rather than my own worst enemy. As a result, life became a lot sweeter and far more pleasant.

I caution you to be careful about what you tell yourself. Also, remember that health, wellness, and fitness are measured by how you feel and how you move, rather than a size or a number. You cannot feel good when you are talking negatively about yourself—no matter what you look like. It is not healthy, nor is it helpful. It's important to be kind to yourself, to give yourself positive messages, and to keep exploring the many opportunities you have to keep yourself *forever fit and flexible*. What I discovered in my own life and through working with others is that when we have a more positive outlook, we become stronger and more confident. Our relationships also get better because the negative people seem to drift away and the positively-charged individuals are attracted to us. With the right mindset, we can truly soar.

chapter three

Building Your Foundation

"Build it … or it will fall."

Everything starts from the bottom up. You absolutely need a solid foundation from which to move. It makes no sense to attempt to strengthen or stretch your body when you are not properly aligned and balanced within your structure. It is like trying to build a house on a faulty foundation. Once you start adding the bricks and mortar, the building is going to collapse in on itself. The same principle applies to our bodies, although they are certainly far more beautiful and spectacular, both in design and function.

There are four building blocks to a solid foundation: structure, core strength, flexibility, and balance. Each one is equally important. Together, they work to support your structure.

However, they need to be addressed in the order in which they are presented for them to be effective. For example, you can't improve your flexibility or your balance if you don't have neutral postural alignment and core strength. Nor can you improve your core strength if you don't have good structural alignment (posture). These components are the pillars that we build upon, much like building a house. You wouldn't think about putting the bricks and mortar in place without first digging the foundation and then building the frame. Each step is equally important and must be done in the proper order to insure a strong, fit, and flexible body. Let's take a brief look at each one and begin to experience them in our bodies.

A solid foundation is the product of a sound structure, and a sound structure is a result of correct postural alignment. Did you notice I didn't say "good" posture? I phrased it that way intentionally, because a lot of us have hang-ups regarding our posture. Most of us have struggled with our posture at some point in our life, and there is a lot of judgment (and even shame or embarrassment) related to our "bad posture." This relates back to the concept of self-image and our belief system. "I have bad posture so I must be a bad person," "I'm not trying hard enough," "I'm lazy," etc. Then, the litany of negative self-talk begins. Instead of putting a label on our posture such as "good" or "bad," we all need to find the neutral alignment of our own individual skeletal structure. This allows us to move easily and effortlessly, rather than try to hold ourselves in unnatural positions that are impossible to hold and, as a result, leave our bodies in pain, dysfunction, and inflexibility.

Here is a simple experiment for you to see if your alignment is in skeletal neutral. As you do what follows, I ask that you also keep a neutral mind and observe. Remember, there is no good or bad here—just observation of what is.

Sit up tall in a position that you believe is good posture. See how long you can stay in this position until you feel fatigue or discomfort and have to let go of it. How long could you sit in that position? Did you feel like you were working hard to stay upright? If so, then you're probably not in neutral. Now, scoot forward on your chair (this works best if you are sitting on a firm surface) until your sit bones (called the ischial tuberosities) are on the edge of the chair. Notice what it's like to sit upright now compared to how you were before. If it feels easier, it's because your spine and your skeletal structure have a solid base in the form of your sit bones and your pelvis. The bones naturally stack themselves up without your muscles having to work overtime to get you in that position and keep you there.

This is a simple way to improve your posture without trying a lot of silly maneuvers that actually make your posture worse instead of better. We will further address the subject of posture in Chapter Six and experiment with several movement lessons to help you find neutral alignment as well as effortless posture.

To help support your foundation and give it strength and stability, we will move on to core strength. The good news is that we are not going to waste our time doing crunches and sit-ups. You have probably already been there and done that. Traditional crunches and sit-ups do not effectively strengthen and shape your core muscles. However, they can cause significant injury to your neck and back, not to mention to your psychological health and well-being.

Here's another little experiment for you to play with. Get down on the floor and do a few crunches. Notice what your abdominal muscles are doing as you crunch up ... are they pulling in or pooching out? How does your neck feel? If you can easily hold the crunch position for a slow count of ten, with no tension in your neck while you pull your abdominals in at the same time, you are most likely doing them correctly. If not, I'm sorry to say that you're wasting your time and risking injury to your neck. You might even be building abdominal muscles that pooch *out* instead of *in*. Yikes!

There is a much easier and more effective way to develop your core, and you may be surprised to discover a technique that is extremely simple and makes a lot more sense than grinding out crunches and sit-ups. We will go into far more detail in Chapter Seven, but until then, sit on the very edge of a firm chair just as you did in the previous paragraph. See if you can find that position where your spine seems to balance easily over your sit bones. Inhale, and as you exhale, gently pull your lower abdominal muscles in and up toward your spine without tilting your pelvis. This action will activate a specific abdominal muscle that is responsible for supporting your spine and stabilizing your pelvis. It also gives you a flatter tummy and a shapely waistline. Have I captured your attention?

Flexibility is another essential component of your foundation. If there is not enough "give" in your structure, it will crack and crumble. When you start to lose flexibility, everything else falls apart as well. Traditional stretches do not always work, and it is not because you are not trying hard enough, not doing them often enough, or are doing them incorrectly. There is a specific physiological explanation for this, which we will discuss in more detail later in the program. For now, though, let's try something to connect you with your flexibility.

Lie down on the floor with one leg resting on the floor and

your knee straight. Bend your other knee, place the foot flat on the floor, and place both hands just below your knee to bring it toward your chest to stretch. Notice how far you can comfortably stretch, including where you might feel tight or restricted. Take a moment to relax the muscles in the front of your hip and see how much further you can go. Were you able to go a little further once you relaxed the front of the hip you were stretching? Unfortunately, sometimes when we stretch our muscles, the soft tissues surrounding the joint tighten up even more to protect the joint from injury. We'll explore this in more detail in Chapter Eight.

Balance is another building block in our foundation and works together closely with flexibility to provide what we refer to as *dynamic stability*. You need to be able to move, as well as to adapt quickly and easily to abrupt changes in your environment, without falling over. To be able to move through these changes, we have to find an internal flow and flexibility instead of a rigid position. Not only does this relate directly to flexibility, it's also associated with posture as well.

Moshe Feldenkrais never used the word "posture." He called it "acture," because we should be able to move at any time, in any direction, and from any position without having to make preparatory adjustments to be able to move. In other words, our bodies and our brains are always ready for action at any split second in time. Not only is it better for your body and your overall health, it is a survival strategy as well. Besides, we are meant and made to move.

Here is another little experiment to try. Stand up as straight and tall as you possibly can, just as you did in the sitting position when we addressed posture. First, notice how long you could hold that position without getting tired or having your muscles begin to cramp. Now imagine that a tiger has suddenly burst through the door of the room you are in with the intention to cause you harm. Yes, that tiger is coming directly toward you, and at a rapid speed. Could you move easily and effortlessly from this position without having to take a few microseconds to make adjustments before you would be able to move to safety? If not, those few microseconds would give the tiger the tactical advantage to make you his lunch.

In this day and age, the chances of a tiger bursting in on you are highly unlikely, but this principle does apply to any situation where you might need to make a quick getaway. So, let's take this a step further. Gently relax or soften your knees. You may notice that you have a bit of movement or slight swaying happening rather than your body being completely still or rigid. You might also notice that your feet connect with the floor more solidly, and you are more grounded and connected with the floor instead of feeling as if you are precariously hovering over it. Take a moment to feel the movement going through you, and once again imagine that tiger bursting in on you. From this position, could you move easily and effortlessly without having to take a few microseconds to make adjustments before you would be able to move to safety? Notice how this stance is different from your previous experiment with your knees locked. Are you able to move more easily now, in any direction, without having to make preparatory adjustments? With this stance, you are more flexible in your ability to move in an environment that is constantly changing, and you are also able to maintain your balance more easily because you are more grounded. We will dive in deeper and play further with balance in Chapter Nine.

I recently met a woman who told me that she'd discovered how many opportunities she had to do her squats just by taking pictures of her young grandson when she was babysitting. Bingo! That's what I'm talking about! She also shared with me how much her legs ached the next day, but in a good way, so she knew that she was getting in a good leg workout. There is a perfect example of the four foundational components in use. Her structure was aligned in a neutral position, allowing her to use her core muscles as she constantly had to change positions to photograph her active grandson. She was able to bend from her hips and knees rather than bend from her back because her postural alignment was in a neutral position, further strengthening her legs, mobilizing her hip joints (flexibility), and saving wear and tear on her spine and back muscles. Since her posture, core strength, and flexibility were in place, she could quickly change her position as she kept her balance. And she managed all of this without having to think about it. Since she was already on the right track, I showed her how to activate her abdominal muscles when she did squats to take his pictures, as well as when she picked him up to further strengthen her core muscles. Through these movements, she was strengthening her legs, her abdominals, and her arms, all while she enjoyed precious time with her grandson. Not only that, she was protecting her back as well.

Even mundane acts such as going to the grocery store, unloading the dishwasher, doing laundry, or simply getting up and down from a chair can offer fantastic opportunities for functional strengthening. You can add additional strengthening exercises as well as physical activities, and you will get a lot more positive effects for your efforts than you ever have before.

chapter four

The Art of Movement

"The basic four will teach you more."

As stated in the introduction, the most significant methods and movement arts that have been influential in developing my *Forever Fit and Flexible* program include Pilates, Feldenkrais, dance, and martial arts. The following is a brief overview of each, along with some of the ways each has impacted my life.

THE POWER OF PILATES

Pilates has been an important part of my life since I first experienced it in 1983. Even after my first lesson, I could feel my spine getting stronger and longer. I felt my abdominal muscles begin to engage in a way I had never felt before. I loved being on the Pilates reformer for many reasons, but mostly because this unique piece of equipment can stretch, strengthen, and sculpt your entire body in just a few sessions. Even when I had no accessibility to classes using the Pilates reformer, I would get on the floor almost every day to do some of the original mat exercises designed by Joseph Pilates. It was when I stopped doing Pilates that I injured my back, and it was gentle Pilates that helped me recover.

When I was a physical therapy student, I sang the praises of Pilates to my classmates, professors, and clinical instructors. Actually, I told anyone who would listen to me about the healing power of this extraordinary method and the man who developed it. I always got the same response: "Well, Pilates is good for dancers, but not really for anyone else." Oh, really? Even as a physical therapy student, I was able to use the principles of Pilates and break down the mat exercises to help my patients achieve their rehabilitation goals.

I remember a time when one of my classmates and I were assigned to a nursing home for a clinical rotation. Carrie was working with a gentleman who I will refer to as "Joe," in honor of Joseph Pilates. Joe had both legs amputated below the knee and was confined to a wheelchair. He was a young man (only fifty), and all he wanted to do was go home to the apartment he shared with his daughter. Unfortunately, Joe was unable to transfer himself from his wheelchair to his bed, bathroom, or the car without the maximum amount of assistance from two people. Unless he could master the ability to move himself from one location to another, which was considered a simple task, he was never going to leave the nursing home.

Carrie worked hard to help Joe learn how to transfer himself so he could go home. She was an excellent student and tried every technique she could think of—with no success. She had him on a strengthening program for his arms and his core muscles, which were already strong, but he still couldn't push himself up from his chair to transfer himself without two people helping him. Finally, out of desperation, she asked me to take a look at him to see if I could help. I tried not to panic because I didn't know what I could possibly do that she hadn't already done. Besides, I knew how much was on the line for Joe, and I felt my own anxiety threaten to spiral out of control.

My first step was for me to watch Joe try to transfer himself. Suddenly my anxiety melted away as I zoomed in on the problem. Actually it was so obvious I was surprised no one else had seen it. Every time Joe pushed his arms against the chair, all of his effort was lost in the area between his shoulder blades. He had no strength in the muscles between his shoulder blades to support the work his arms were doing. I immediately thought of a Pilates mat exercise that would help.

The exercise is called "The Single Leg Kick," and in its original form wasn't appropriate for him. However, I believed that one of the basic principles behind the exercise was crucial to helping Joe learn how to transfer himself. I modified the "Single Leg Kick" to be done as Joe sat on a mat in the physical therapy gym with a large exercise ball in front of him to press his forearms against while he pulled his elbows in toward his waist to activate the muscles he needed to connect with. I made a few other modifications so that even Joseph Pilates himself wouldn't have recognized it as one of his original exercises. I am sure, though, that he would have understood what I was after and applauded my thought process behind it.

That one exercise certainly did the trick. By the end of one week, Joe was able to push himself up and get his body just a few inches off the seat of his chair. By the end of the second week, he was able to transfer himself with minimal help from one person. By the end of the third week, he was able to transfer himself independently and was discharged from the nursing home. Everyone thought I was a genius, but I knew better. I was just the messenger; Joseph Pilates was the mastermind, and the patient was the one who did all the heavy lifting, so to speak.

Pilates enjoyed quite a boom of popularity several years ago and was advertised as a "new" form of exercise. In reality, Joseph H. Pilates founded his method almost one hundred years ago.

Joseph Pilates was a small, sickly child who suffered from asthma and rickets, a bone disorder caused by a lack of Vitamin D, resulting in deformities and fractures. Due to his small stature and slight build, he was often the target of the neighborhood bullies. His fear of tuberculosis as well as his popularity with the bullies prompted him to pursue a life of health and fitness.

Joseph Pilates began a bodybuilding program at an early age, developing such a fit and muscular physique that by the time he was fourteen years old he was being used as a model for anatomy charts. He continued his incredible journey into physical fitness and became an accomplished gymnast, boxer, skier, and acrobat. This small, sickly child actually began to earn a living performing as an acrobat as well as teaching physical fitness and self-defense. What an amazing story!

Joseph Pilates was performing in a circus as an acrobat in England in 1912, when World War I broke out. As a German national, he was placed in an internment camp for the duration of the war. During that time, Joseph Pilates further expanded on his ideas of health, wellness, and fitness, even leading exercise classes for his fellow inmates to help them survive and thrive in the deplorable conditions of the internment camp. His ideas and experimentation eventually evolved into The Pilates Method that we know today.

Pilates truly embodies the mind-body connection that we talked about in Chapter One, by engaging your attention and awareness of every exercise you do. This thoughtful attention to each exercise helps you stretch, strengthen, and re-shape your entire body far more quickly than any traditional exercise program. Pilates and the level of awareness that it cultivates also help you prevent and recover from injuries while you strengthen your core, and improve your posture, balance, and flexibility at the same time.

There are six basic universally-accepted principles of Pilates: concentration, control, centering, flowing movement, precision of movement, and breathing. Each of these principles can help you in your own journey to fitness and flexibility, so it's important to keep them in mind as you create your *Forever Fit and Flexible* program. Let's take a look at each principle individually.

Concentration: When you use your attention to concentrate on your physical movements as well as the sensations you experience as you do them, you get the maximum benefit out of each and every exercise or movement pattern. It sounds exhausting, and it does take some time and energy at first, but the more you practice concentrating, the easier it gets. This depth of concentration also alerts you to warning signals—that you might be doing something incorrectly or are in jeopardy of injuring yourself. As I've experienced many times in my life, most injuries are self-induced as well as preventable.

Control: All movements must be done with absolute control. There is no room for sloppy, forced, or haphazard movements. You move with control and fire up more muscle fibers as well as the individual nerve endings that innervate them, which results in the development of more strength and tone from every Pilates exercise in less time and less effort than traditional exercise. As an added bonus, control also keeps you from injuring yourself.

Centering: In Pilates, centering is a term that refers to a starting place from where all movement begins. It is the area of your body from the bottom of your ribs to the wings on each side of your pelvis and circles around your back much like an internal girdle or corset, sometimes called core strength. Pilates focuses on simultaneously firming, stretching, and strengthening our center, which supports our spine and our pelvis to prevent or reverse low back pain and injuries. These muscles must be engaged to effectively complete all exercises and achieve the wonderful results of a well-developed center, which include a smaller waist, flatter belly, and better posture.

I can't help but feel annoyed when I see advertisements on how to get rid of "belly fat" by buying certain products or having procedures done. By strengthening your center, you will not have belly fat—you'll have muscles instead, and you'll love the way you look.

Flowing movement: In Pilates, you are instructed to work within the limits of your abilities and not push beyond them to the point where you feel stress or strain. By moving with a continuous flow, you can easily identify these limitations and gently begin to work beyond them without injuring yourself. Abrupt ballistic actions are a great way to get hurt, which was driven home for me when I yanked myself up on the ballet barre and tore my triceps. All movement should flow out from a strong center, which is also associated with control. Every exercise begins by activating your center and allowing every movement to effortlessly flow outward from this point. This reinforces the strength of your center and allows for greater ease and freedom of movement as well increasing the range of motion in all of your joints without stress or strain.

Precision of movement: Precision of movement is also a close partner of control. It is the accuracy of each component of every movement that helps to engage your mind and give you the fantastic results that Pilates has to offer. Every detail of each exercise is crucial, even down to the position and placement of your hands and feet. Precision can also be considered a form of fine-tuning of our body's motor skills, and works in conjunction with concentration. This precision and accuracy of movement has a deep physiologic effect on muscle tissue by recruiting more individual muscle fibers and the nerve fibers that innervate them, resulting in the ultimate neuromuscular re-patterning.

Breathing: Breathing should be a no-brainer, but it is amazing how often we hold our breath, especially when we are doing physical activities that we find difficult or challenging. The rhythm of our breath also helps us perform more challenging movements without stress or strain. The breathing should be smooth and natural, and in rhythm with your movements, to assist with the flowing movement and control of each exercise. Holding our breath actually makes movement difficult and almost impossible, where a slow, smooth exhale helps make movement easier. And it helps activate our lower abdominal muscles.

Take a few minutes right now to think about these six principles. This is your first lesson in training your awareness.

By incorporating these principles into all of your movements and exercises, your body and your brain will work together to help you achieve amazing results in a relatively short time. Indeed, the depth of activation of your nerves and muscles is what makes Pilates so effective in changing the shape and tone of your entire body. The result is a long, lean, muscular physique, along with improved posture and core strength. Joseph Pilates would often repeat a quote from Friedrich von Schiller, "It is the mind itself which shapes the body."[1] Think of the power behind that statement. It also makes it pretty clear why my client's weight loss group failed so completely. Joseph Pilates himself was fond of saying, "With Pilates, you are in control of your body, not at its mercy."[2] Pilates also frequently said that long after he was gone, people would say he had been years ahead of his time. He was right about that!

Pilates exercises can either be done on the floor (referred to as mat work) or by using equipment that Joseph Pilates designed himself. Although the mat exercises can be incredibly effective, they are also very challenging and must be approached with caution. It is easy to injure yourself doing the mat exercises if you don't have a strong sense of body awareness or if you have any pre-existing injuries. However, once you develop good core strength as well as greater self-awareness, the mat work is a fantastic option for a thorough and efficient workout. It has the distinct advantage of being portable and can be done anywhere and at any time. You do not need special equipment or even weights to do an effective Pilates mat workout.

1. The Pilates Method of Physical and Mental Conditioning by Philip Friedman and Gail Eisen, Doubleday & Company, 1980

2. The Pilates Method of Physical and Mental Conditioning by Philip Friedman and Gail Eisen, Doubleday & Company, 1980

The most common and well-known piece of Pilates equipment was named "The Universal Reformer" by Joseph Pilates, and is referred to today simply as "The Reformer." Although the reformer looks formidable, it is a wonderful tool to safely and effectively help people who are injured, in chronic pain, or have other physical challenges, strengthen their core, lengthen their spine, improve their posture, and learn how to move without pain. On the other hand, the same piece of equipment can be utilized to challenge individuals who are quite fit and want to improve and increase their level of conditioning. Even professional athletes and dancers can use the reformer to fine tune their skills and give them a competitive edge. The original reformer was created so efficiently by Joseph Pilates that the only components that have changed from his original design are the materials used to build them. The man was a genius.

Joseph Pilates did not teach large group classes like the ones that are popular today. He only worked with individual clients in private sessions to provide them with the proper amount of attention to help them change their physique and address their specific needs and concerns. It is interesting to note that in the early days of Joseph Pilates, his program was one of the best kept secrets among professional dancers and other performing artists. They all flocked to his small studio in Manhattan, once they discovered that his techniques could help them improve their strength and stamina. They found his method invaluable in helping them stay healthy and injury free under the grueling demands of their careers.

One final point I would like to make regarding Pilates. It was after I stopped practicing Pilates and attending weekly Pilates classes that my insidious onset of low back pain came creeping in, eventually rendering me incapacitated. I am convinced that if I hadn't stopped doing Pilates I never would have hurt my back. I continue to practice Pilates every single day, but not in the traditional sense of attending classes or getting on my reformer for a workout. Rather, I incorporate the basic principles of Pilates every day, in everything I do. I have no desire to ever repeat the experience of being a chronic pain patient again, at least not if I can help it—and Pilates is definitely here to help.

MOVEMENT IS LIFE – THE FELDENKRAIS METHOD®

I had my first experience with Feldenkrais in the spring of 2000, when I took a three-day Feldenkrais workshop for dancers. I wasn't exactly sure what the method was all about, but by the end of those three days I felt better than I had in years. My legs felt longer, my hips and my back felt looser, and my mood was lighter. This general feeling of well-being persisted for the next several weeks, and I began taking weekly Feldenkrais group classes from a local practitioner. I still wasn't sure what was happening to create this incredible new sense of vitality, but I did know that I liked how I was feeling. I also knew I had to become a practitioner and add this skillset to my list of services, not only to help my clients but to help me in my life as well.

Unlike Pilates, The Feldenkrais Method® is not a system of exercise, although it is a method of movement. You might say that Feldenkrais is a highly sophisticated form of movement therapy, but it is more accurate to call it a method of movement re-education based on the process of learning and self-discovery. I know, it sounds like a mouthful as well as a bit of *New-Age woo-woo*. Let me assure you, though, that it is not.

Feldenkrais is based on the scientific principle of neuro-plasticity, which simply means that we are capable of learning new patterns and changing the way we move, sense, think, and feel during the entire course of our lifetime. We'll go into more detail a little later, but first allow me to introduce you to the man behind the method, Moshe Feldenkrais.

In contrast to Joseph Pilates, Moshe Feldenkrais was a very healthy and robust individual who enjoyed a variety of physical activities from a young age, including soccer and judo. However, just as Pilates founded his method out of his own personal adversity, Feldenkrais developed his unique formula for movement from his own need to heal after a devastating knee injury, which he incurred while playing soccer. Although his knee seemed to heal, he repeatedly re-injured it, oftentimes as a result of doing nothing more strenuous than stepping off a curb.

After seeking help from multiple physicians, as well as trying various types of physical rehabilitation, he was advised that surgery was the only option available to him. He was also informed that the chance of surgery being successful was about fifty-fifty. Feldenkrais didn't even bother to find out what the surgeon's definition of "successful" was, since he wasn't willing to accept the odds. Instead of surgery or continuing other therapies (which weren't working anyway), he decided to try to fix his knee himself. Through a process of using his mindful awareness, Feldenkrais noticed that certain movements and positions of his leg made his knee feel much stronger, more stable, and pain free. Conversely, he noticed how other positions and movement patterns had the opposite effect, making his knee feel weak, unstable, and painful. He continued the process of gentle movement explorations until his knee injury was completely healed.

Somehow, his story of self-healing spread through his neighborhood and other people suffering with knee problems sought out his help. The more people he helped, the more he learned, and the more his methodology unfolded and became what it is now. I can't help but wonder what might have happened if Moshe Feldenkrais had opted to go ahead with the surgery. With today's modern technology and arthroscopic procedures, knee surgery is relatively easy to recover from and has an extremely high success rate. However, during the 1930s and 1940s it was much more complicated with far different results. The standing joke among the Feldenkrais community is that if arthroscopic surgery had been around during Moshe's time, we would not have the Feldenkrais Method® today.

From his own experimentation, Moshe Feldenkrais created an incredibly powerful system of self-learning through movement by cultivating consciousness with movement patterns. What developed is a gentle but powerful process of self-education. The learning takes place deep in our nervous system, which allows us to gently interrupt patterns of movement that may be causing pain, stress, joint dysfunction, immobility, or other issues that interfere with our quality of life.

Although Feldenkrais is considered a therapeutic modality, it is different from traditional therapies because there is no "protocol" or predetermined list of exercises. Instead, the focus is on exploring new patterns of movement through our own personal experience. It is a method where we get to discover for ourselves how to move without pain, strain, stress, and effort. In traditional therapies, the emphasis is placed on the practitioner "fixing the patient" or "correcting the problem." In Feldenkrais, the focus is placed on paying attention to ourselves and the quality of our movement. There is no good or bad, right or wrong, better or worse; just opportunities to learn. You get to find what you could do, instead of having someone tell you what you should or must do. It is a very empowering experience.

Unlike the Pilates Method, Feldenkrais does not have specific orthodox principles to follow, but it does have one major cardinal rule, which is that you have to be able to make yourself comfortable for it to be effective. When we experience pain or discomfort, our nervous system is focused on the sense of unease and isn't able to attend to the new sensations going through us. For many of us, just the idea of making ourselves comfortable is a novel idea. It might even seem a bit self-indulgent, especially in our "no pain no gain" mentality. Think about the times you decided to push through the pain and keep going. How did that work out for you? The approach with Feldenkrais is far more forgiving, and the results are incredible.

Another concept that makes Feldenkrais unique is that it focuses on moving from our skeleton rather than pushing from our muscles. It is our skeletal structure that supports us; it is our bones and our joints that propel us through space; and it is our brain and our nervous system that put it all together to create movement. Our muscles contract and relax according to the messages they receive from our nervous system. It is a completely different approach to movement, but the outcome is that our bodies are able to move easily and effortlessly, without aches, pains, stress, and strain. What is even more remarkable is that our muscles actually get stronger and more toned, in spite of the fact that we are not trying to work them. Our joints also become looser and our spines become longer.

Moshe used to say that his method "made the impossible possible, the possible easy, and the easy effortless." Feldenkrais just makes everything easier, and better. However, *better* isn't a word you will hear in a Feldenkrais session, since the key to allowing our nervous system to change is to "talk" to it in a powerful but gentle way, through movement and without the constraints of judging the process. It's incredibly liberating.

There are two types of Feldenkrais lessons: Awareness Through Movement® lessons and Functional Integration® lessons. Awareness Through Movement classes are movement explorations developed by Moshe Feldenkrais. These lessons are group classes, where your practitioner verbally guides the class through specific movement patterns. You are encouraged to move slowly, at your own pace and timing, to allow your body and your brain the opportunity to explore new patterns of movement. You get to discover for yourself what you *could* do, instead of having someone else telling you what you *should* do.

Functional Integration lessons are individual, private sessions where your practitioner gently takes you through a series of movements based on your individual needs or limitations. Chronic pain and injuries are often a result of faulty movement patterns that cause destructive forces through your body. During Functional Integration lessons, these faulty movement patterns are gently interrupted and new movement patterns are introduced. These "hands-on" lessons capture your body's own ability to correct your structural alignment. The result is a decrease in aches and pains and a greater capacity to move more easily and to participate in the activities you enjoy. Additionally, both Awareness Through Movement lessons and Functional Integration lessons increase your level of energy and vitality.

Feldenkrais also gives you a greater sense of self-confidence. Moshe Feldenkrais used to say, "What I'm after isn't flexible bodies, it is flexible brains. What I'm after is to restore each person to his human dignity."[3] Isn't that a lovely philosophy to live by?

Just like Joseph Pilates, Moshe Feldenkrais was years ahead of his time regarding his understanding of the human body and the human nervous system. It has only been in the past twenty years that neuroscientists have discovered that neuroplasticity is present at every age and in every stage of life. Prior to that time, it was believed that this natural miracle disappeared at about the age of fourteen.

Feldenkrais isn't limited to helping people eliminate pain and move better. It is a valuable tool to help people with a variety of developmental or neurological disorders discover a much higher level of function. Athletes and performing artists alike can enjoy a greater level of skill with much less effort, resulting in a higher level of performance and giving them a competitive edge.

Taylor, my niece, is an outstanding volleyball player. But when she started really upping her game, she began to experience low back pain during volleyball practice, especially when she served the ball. When she reported it to one of her coaches, the coach told Taylor that it was common for girls to have back pain with volleyball, and it might go away if she got stronger and worked harder. That made no sense to me, since no one should have back pain at the age of thirteen. Besides, she was already strong enough and certainly worked hard enough. I had Taylor show me how she served the ball and immediately saw what was happening to cause her back pain. I gave her a few tips to correct her positioning when she served the ball. Not only did her back pain disappear, her

3. Quote from Tubegator Famous Quotes at quotes.tubegator.com

serve got even more powerful. Score one for Feldenkrais! I even gave my husband tips on how to improve his golf swing, something that he was a little resistant to hear since I have never held a golf club in my life and know nothing about the game. My father was an avid golfer and loved hearing that story. My dad even let me do Feldenkrais with him at the end of his life to help him get back on the golf course and enjoy a few more games with his buddies before he died. What an honor for me, and what a wonderful memory.

As for myself, the Feldenkrais Method® changed my life. It lengthened my legs, strengthened my spine, loosened my hips, and opened my heart. It made everything in life easier and effortless. Feldenkrais also helped me get rid of chronic headaches, neck pain, stress, and fatigue. It even helped me recover from the nightmare of post-traumatic stress. As one of my clients told me, "Feldenkrais is like finding freedom! Sweet freedom!" She's right; Feldenkrais gives you the freedom to be yourself. Feldenkrais is magic, but as you now know, there is solid science behind that magic.

DANCE YOUR WAY TO BETTER HEALTH

Regardless of the style of dance you practice or may be interested in, dance is the motherlode for fitness, flexibility, and health. It doesn't matter if you are a classical dancer or a closet dancer—nothing beats the benefits of dance. For me personally, I absolutely love the grueling regimen and relentless discipline of a professional level ballet class, as long as I'm not tearing my triceps. Some people prefer the gliding elegance of ballroom dance, while others are devoted tap dancers. I can appreciate their passion for tap, because I still remember the joy of banging those shoes against a hardwood dance floor, joined by the chaotic cacophony of a dozen other preschoolers. I have a few clients who swear by Zumba, while others simply turn on the music, lower their blinds, and freestyle to their heart's content in the privacy of their own home. Have you ever heard the saying, "Dance like no one is watching"? That's what they do, and they love it. The point is: you can dance in any style, at any time, and at any age.

When I was a physical therapy student, we took a field trip to a local senior center. It was a lovely recreation center, filled to capacity with white-haired senior citizens who had gathered together to play cards, pool, and backgammon, to read and enjoy a variety of relaxing activities.

Our last stop was the gym, where another group was rehearsing a tap routine in preparation for an upcoming performance. They were just about to take it from the top when we walked in, and we were graciously invited to watch. There were at least ten women, one token man, and they were amazing! One dancer sat in a chair in the center of the group while her fellow dancers tapped up a storm around her. Just when I thought it couldn't get any better, the dancers stepped off to the side and the woman on the chair began to move. My jaw dropped, and my classmates, who were much younger than me, almost hit the floor.

This woman moved from her chair in a most seductive and alluring manner, making us a captive and most appreciative audience. Not only was she a beautiful dancer, she had the best legs I have ever seen, and she was downright sexy. The other dancers joined her, and they came together for a spectacular finale. I had tears in my eyes as my classmates had to forcibly remove me from the gym. I so desperately wanted to stay with them and have that remarkable lady teach me everything she knew. I was ready to throw my education and my physical therapy career away with both hands and pick up a pair of tap shoes to join her. Instead, I let my study buddies take me away to dream of the day when I would dance again rather than sit on my butt for fourteen interminable hours a day.

Dance is great exercise, and it's so much fun that it doesn't seem like work at all. Sometimes I even forget that I'm working out. The last time I saw a doctor, he asked me what type of exercise I did. I didn't know what to say because I don't exercise, which is a little embarrassing since I am a physical therapist. After all, I don't go to the gym, I don't run, I don't do a walking program, and I don't do anything that is usually defined as "exercise." I was stumped. Finally, I did a mental head smack. *That's right, I dance!* Relieved, I answered, "I'm a dancer." He said, "How nice. Ballroom?" I replied, "No, ballet." He almost fell off his chair. I guess he hadn't come across many fifty-plus-year-old ballet dancers in his practice. I can't imagine what his reaction would be if I ever return to him and tell him I started pole dancing last year. Believe it or not, I am not the only lady over fifty in ballet class, nor am I the only one at the pole either.

There are many different forms of dance, and you are never too old to try them, no matter what anyone else says, thinks, or tries to tell you to the contrary. Dance has also always been used as a form of healing as well as self-expression. It has been an important part of human civilization since the beginning of time, as part of religious ceremonies, rituals, celebrations, and entertainment. Any style of dance is fantastic exercise for your body, mind, and spirit. It is the panacea that leads to good health, and there are multiple benefits of dance besides the combined effects of socialization and improved physical fitness.

Dance helps you increase your metabolism and control your weight while you simultaneously strengthen your entire body and improve your posture, balance, and flexibility. Additional physical benefits include greater endurance, stamina, and coordination. The benefits go beyond the physical, with positive psychological effects, including a decrease in stress and anxiety. It almost sounds too good to be true. However, the news about the health benefits of dance get even better.

Recent studies have revealed the most extraordinary health benefit gained through any style of dance—it improves brain function. The combined effort of learning and remembering new dance steps while you challenge your balance and coordination as you listen to music stimulates your brain and awakens your nervous system. The result is an increase in memory and mental function, spatial orientation, and peripheral vision. That certainly should be enough to convince you to put on your dancing shoes!

Finally, there is nothing that can quite compare to the social aspect of dance and the exhilaration of getting together with a group of people who share a passion with you. One of the many reasons why I still go to ballet class is because it's fantastic girlfriend time, and a lot of us have supported each other through a variety of life's traumas and triumphs over the past thirty years. But the number one reason I dance is simply because it fills my heart with joy. I just couldn't imagine saying that about a trip to the gym. Could you?

THE TRUTH ABOUT MARTIAL ARTS

My father began his study of karate when he was in his early forties. By that time, I had yet another sister. I guess after having five daughters my dad figured he needed to have a solid set of skills to protect them. For years he tried to get me and my sisters to go to the gym to train with him, but we all turned deaf ears to his persuasive arguments. Imagine his surprise (and everyone else's) when I began my martial arts training at the age of forty-seven. He actually was able to watch me work out when I was a yellow belt, and we had many interesting conversations regarding the physical and spiritual elements of martial arts. It's like being a member of an exclusive club where only the members fully understand how martial arts training can change a person's life. I am pleased to say that my father lived long enough to see me earn my third degree brown belt.

Martial arts have been around for thousands of years. The ability for man to be able to protect himself, his family, and his tribe have been paramount to his very survival. To be able to succeed in combat, mock battles were simulated to practice defense tactics against a variety of life-threatening situations; from individuals, warring tribes, and natural predators. These mock battles were the earliest form of martial arts practices. They were designed to improve the attention, reflexes, strength, and ability of the warrior to respond appropriately to any circumstance at any moment.

One of the greatest misconceptions about martial arts is that they are all based on the principle of fighting and/or warfare. Although that was how the study of martial arts began, in reality nothing could be further from the truth. Of course, studying a martial art does give you the tools you need to be able to protect yourself, but the purpose is not to promote violence. Martial arts are about movement, survival, and self-defense; but they are also about pursuing peace and harmony through training your body, mind, and spirit.

Martial arts training provides fabulous exercise to strengthen your body, improve your general conditioning, increase stamina, and build endurance. There is also a tremendous amount of concentration and brain power involved in studying any type of martial art, resulting in improved mental focus and acuity. Individuals who train in martial arts have a reputation for experiencing tremendous anti-aging benefits due to the physical and mental strengthening that develops from training. The practice of slow, controlled movements, combined with the constant weight shifting and change of directions, develops sharper reflexes and quicker responses. Aging martial artists often move better and think more clearly than people much younger than they.

Another benefit of martial arts is a little more difficult to measure. It is called spirit, and it is a combination of values and character traits, such as respect, discipline, and self-control. Martial arts are also a wonderful way to relieve stress and frustration. They provide a healthy alternative for expressing negative feelings rather than turning them inward and causing illness. They also help you learn how to choose your battles and how to walk away from a potentially volatile situation before it implodes on you.

There are two basic styles of martial arts, which are categorized as "hard styles" and "soft styles." The hard styles involve meeting force with force against an attacker with powerful strikes and kicks to defeat them. Karate and Tae Kwan Do are examples of the hard styles of martial arts. The soft styles of martial arts focus more on internal power and can be considered a form of moving meditation. Tai Chi is an example of a soft style martial art. If you watch a group of students performing their Tai Chi patterns, it looks like they are barely moving and cannot possibly be working very hard. In reality, moving that slowly through the patterns takes an incredible amount of balance and concentration. It is an art form that can be done in a large group or on your own at home.

Just like Pilates mat exercises, the portability of a Tai Chi practice is very appealing. Also, it is important to note that it typically does not include sparring. However, when it does, the techniques are based more on using leverage rather than muscular tension and force. That alone makes it more appealing to people over fifty, who would like to study a martial art but do not want to take the risk of getting injured by an overly enthusiastic training partner. Tai Chi is an excellent choice for the over-fifty population and a practice that can keep you healthy and fit as you age, as the following story illustrates.

A few years ago I worked part-time in a subacute rehabilitation center, which is an inpatient facility that provides physical and occupational therapy to patients who are unable to tolerate the intense therapy they would receive in a rehabilitation center. One afternoon, I saw an elderly gentleman moving in the courtyard behind the therapy gym. I stopped and watched him as he moved gracefully and effortlessly through a series of intricate movement patterns. After about twenty minutes, he stopped, bent down, picked up a tennis ball, and began playing with the chocolate lab puppy that also doubled as a therapy dog for the facility. I noticed two of my colleagues watching him and smiling at each other.

I asked them who he was, and which patient he was visiting. They informed me that this remarkable gentleman was not a visitor; he was a patient. Every day they watched him go outside to practice his Tai Chi. Of course, that was after he made his own bed, took his shower, had his breakfast, and was appropriately dressed and groomed for the day. I was amazed, and I asked them what he was doing at the rehabilitation center, since he certainly didn't appear to need any help. Indeed, he looked like he was in better shape than most of the staff members. One of the therapists replied, "He checked himself into the center because he felt he needed a tune up to increase his strength. He wants to celebrate his 100th birthday next week in style." I am not saying that his incredible health and vitality was solely attributed to his Tai Chi practice, but it certainly does make you wonder.

The most basic and valuable skill that the beginning martial arts student learns is how to get out of the way of an attack. This can translate into a valuable life skill, both on and off of the mat. As you probably already know at this point in your life, life is full of "hits" and none of us get through life without receiving our fair share of them. The principles of martial arts can be applied to every challenging or threatening situation in life, besides physical attacks. Martial arts give you the ability to handle these situations with composure under pressure. They also teach you how to choose your battles. Additionally, there is a powerful healing energy that exists in martial arts. Consequently, many people have been able to recover from physical and emotional challenges through training.

Martial arts are based on the principle of lifelong learning. People often ask me why I still train, since I have already earned my black belt. The truth is a martial artist never really reaches the end. Each step is a new beginning and a new opportunity to learn more about yourself and your art. It is a beautiful journey of self-growth, and it is also another reason why martial artists have a youthful energy and vitality, regardless of their age or the amount of years they've invested in their training. In addition, martial artists develop an incredible sense of peace, calm, and serenity in knowing that they have the ability to protect themselves, no matter what is coming at them.

Pilates, Feldenkrais, dance, and martial arts all share a few common basic principles that make them extremely effective for helping you remain *fit and flexible*. All of them focus on movement as an art form, rather than mindless movement or exercise with no purpose or passion behind it. Each one of these artistic movement methods fully engages your body, mind, and spirit to improve the caliber of your movement and the quality of your life. If you can apply these same basic principles to the movement lessons in this book, as well as in all of your physical activities, you will be amazed at the results. There is nothing magical about these principles—just the magic of what evolves when you pay attention to yourself and how you move.

There are other forms of movement arts that might pique your interest and curiosity, and I encourage you to research any (or all) of them that may appeal to you. The most important point to remember is that you need to keep moving, both literally and figuratively, in every aspect of life. The key is to make it as interesting, pleasurable, and fun as possible. In the *Forever Fit and Flexible* program, the fundamental principles start with fun.

chapter five

Fundamental Principles

"Putting the fun in fun-damental."

The journey to fitness and flexibility can be challenging, but it can also be fun and exciting, as long as you approach it that way. If you look at it with all the enthusiasm of a root canal, it will probably be a bit painful. However, if you begin the journey with a sense of interest, curiosity, and a spirit of playfulness, it will be a lot more appealing. Each step in the journey presents a new challenge and represents a new milestone for you to accomplish. I like to imagine that I am my own personal private detective, discovering clues along the way that lead me to the most effective tools to stay fit and healthy. It is a continuous process, and we are all works in progress.

I must admit that there are still times when I fall flat on my face. I take that as a pretty clear message that I might be doing something wrong. So, after I pick myself up and shake myself off, I put on my detective hat to find the missing clues that might be tripping me up. I review all the steps and then tweak my program to help me get back on the right track again. I encourage you to do the same. After all, you know yourself better than anyone. Don't feel like you have to follow the crowd and do what everyone else is doing. Where's the sport in that? I do encourage you, however, to keep the following basic fundamental principles in mind as you move forward through the program:

1. Each and every movement has a *purpose*. Make each movement count and look for the little micro-movements along the way. Those small, intrinsic micro-movements are rich with information to help you change your body and the way you move.

2. Each and every moment in time deserves its own *attention*. Do not rush through the movement patterns; instead, take your time to pay focused attention to yourself and fully experience each part of every movement lesson.

3. Focus on the *quality* of every movement rather than the quantity or the range of movement. Less is more; be more interested in how the movement patterns *feel* rather than how they *look*.

4. Move *slowly*, slower than you have ever moved before. The slower you move, and the smaller the movements, the more you will be able to feel and sense the changes in yourself—likewise, the faster you will get results. Small changes last longer and have the most powerful effect.

5. Take frequent rests, even though you may feel like you are not doing any work at all and do not need a rest. You do need to rest your attention and also allow time for your mind and body to integrate the changes you experience.

6. Allow at least fifteen minutes of uninterrupted time in a *quiet* environment to do each movement lesson. This means turning off all electrical devices and eliminating all possible distractions, including cell phones, spouses, children, and the family pet.

7. Make yourself *comfortable* as you go through the lessons. "No pain, no gain" has absolutely no role in this program, neither does "just do it." Always work within a comfortable and easy range of motion. Put your focus on the process rather than the end result. The results will come.

8. Tell yourself you can get there. What we *believe* is what we become, and if you give yourself positive messages you will get positive results. If you can dream it, you can do it. Imagine yourself as a strong, fit, and flexible person. Yes … it does work!

There is one other concept to consider as we move forward into the movement lessons. I realize that you might be a visual learner, and the instructions for the movement lessons that follow are presented in the written format. No matter what type of learner you are, here are a few suggestions to help you understand, interpret, and practice the movements. They will also aid you in receiving the maximum benefit from each movement:

First, read the instructions for each separate movement lesson. Next, sit back in your chair, close your eyes, and take a few deep breaths. Then, imagine yourself going through each of the movement patterns. In your own imagination, see yourself doing the exercise. Imagine the sensations going through you as you slowly perform each movement. Finally, open your eyes and read the instructions one more time.

Visualization is a powerful tool to help you access the pathways in your brain that are responsible for successful completion of each movement. It "lights up" your nervous system, captures its attention, and can actually help you achieve results more quickly than when you focus solely on the written instructions. Professional athletes and performing artists have used the highly effective power of visualization for years to improve their performance on the field and on the stage. They continue to practice it because it works for them. It will work for you, too!

To complement the practice of visualization, I highly recommend that you record your observations and experiences as you work through each chapter. This will help you create and fine-tune your own *Forever Fit and Flexible* program. You can document any challenges you face with each topic addressed in the chapter, what individual movement lessons, or parts of the lessons, you felt were most beneficial to you, and what other outside activities you might pursue to help overcome any obstacles and enhance your progress. This interactive approach makes your program uniquely your own and gives you the opportunity to use your imagination rather than slavishly follow someone else's directive. You will also have a great point of reference to return to and track your improvement. Remember to try recording the movement lessons and feel free to add key words or modifications to help you get the most out of every movement.

PART TWO

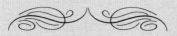

The Program

chapter six

Posture

"You're no slouch, at least not in my book."

Healthy posture is essential to our health, wellness, fitness, and flexibility. Your posture and how you carry yourself are the first things people notice about you, even from a distance. People pay attention to your posture more than you think they do, and it leaves a lasting first impression.

The way you stand, walk, and move communicates to the world how you feel about yourself and what kind of a day you are having. For example, when I first began my martial arts training, I was going through a really bad rough patch in my life, although very few people realized it. I was so skilled at hiding my feelings and was quite a good little actress when the situation warranted, so even my closest friends didn't realize what I was going through. However, my Sensei always knew when I was having an exceptionally bad day. He could see a slight, subtle shift in my posture that nobody else noticed. Sensei detected it because watching people and reading their body language is something he has practiced for years. He told me that I could fool almost anybody, but I would never be able to fool him.

The term "poor posture" is typically associated with a slumped spine, rounded shoulders, and a forward head position. This posture makes you appear timid, tired, and aged. "Good posture" usually refers to someone who stands with a straight spine, shoulders back, and their head lifted. This posture helps you look confident, energetic, and youthful.

In my mind's eye I can see you squirming uncomfortably in your chair as you read these words. You may even be trying to sit up straight by employing a few silly maneuvers that you may have been told over the years constitute "good posture." Unfortunately, a lot of what we've been told, or taught, is wrong. As a matter of fact, there are many misconceptions regarding posture and a great deal of misinformation floating around out there.

One of the most common myths is that our posture naturally deteriorates as we get older and there is absolutely nothing we can do about it. I once read an article, written by experts in their field, which proclaimed that getting shorter was a normal part of the aging process. The article stated that this process begins at the age of thirty. Furthermore, we will lose one-half to three-quarters of an inch with each consecutive decade of life. That means that if I were to fall in line with this prediction, I should be at least two inches shorter than I am now. However, I have not lost a centimeter, let alone an inch.

Apparently the experts are wrong, or I didn't get the memo that I was supposed to start shrinking, and when. In reality, we do lose some of the thickness of our vertebral discs as we mature, but we do not have to lose that much height. We can prevent the loss of height by staying active and engaging in activities that lengthen our spine and improve our posture.

My ballet master had beautiful posture his entire life, until he passed away at the age of eighty-one. He did admit that he had to work a little harder to be more aware of his posture as he got older, and he certainly did an excellent job of it. Of course, as a lifelong dancer, he understood the mechanics of posture as well as his structural alignment, which he used to his advantage.

I have an aunt who is eighty-seven. She has lovely posture and continues to move, and bowl, in a manner that looks graceful and effortless. Yes, she is a bowler, and she continues to excel at it, even at eighty-seven. I honestly do not think she makes a conscious effort to work on her posture, but somewhere deep in her subconscious she knows that her posture is an important component of her skill level. If she allowed her posture to deteriorate, her game would deteriorate as well. Of course, that just wouldn't be acceptable to her. And, that woman sure can bowl!

Another common myth about ideal structural alignment (often referred to as "good posture") is that "military posture" is often regarded as the gold standard for posture. However, the gold standard is tarnished. Try this little experiment based on the requirements for military posture. Stand tall and pull your shoulders back, push out your chest, suck in your stomach, and pinch your buttocks together. How does that feel? Are you able to breathe easily? How long do you think you could maintain that posture? Finally, if that imaginary tiger came bursting into the room, could you move without having to first make some preparatory adjustments? As you may have discovered, this posture is a rigid, stiff, unyielding position that makes it difficult to breathe, let alone move. The stance is unnatural, and our muscles have to work overtime to maintain it. The result is muscle imbalances, back, neck and shoulder pain, joint deterioration, fatigue, and a progressive decline in structural alignment. So much for military posture!

Healthy posture is not "good"—it is effortless. No, this isn't a typo, it's the truth. Posture is not good, bad, or otherwise. It is simply a neutral structural alignment that supports you in an easy, effortless, and even elegant way. Contrary to popular belief, it is not our muscles that support us in the upright position—it is our skeletal structure. Our spine and skeleton are beautifully designed to direct the forces of gravity through us in an easy and effortless manner. When your structure is organized in this natural (or neutral) alignment, your muscles maintain the proper tone and balance. You not only stand and walk more comfortably, but you also have more energy and endurance. You have better standing and dynamic balance, because your center of gravity is directly over your base of support. In addition, your bones become stronger due to the correct line of stress placed on them in weight-bearing activities. You even stand taller, look longer and leaner, and you breathe better.

Here is even more good news: you don't have to suck in your stomach. When you are standing in proper alignment, your abdominal muscles automatically engage. As a result, your abdominal muscles will become stronger, your tummy will become flatter, and your waistline will get smaller. As an added bonus, neutral posture is graceful and elegant, as well as effortless. Neutral posture allows for constant movement and change within your external and internal environment, without unnecessary effort. Besides, it makes you look more youthful. Who wouldn't want that?

On the other hand, there are many detrimental effects on our body that can result from a faulty skeletal structure (or less than neutral posture). The laundry list of potential health problems include: bone loss, osteoporosis, impaired balance, fractures, heart problems, and respiratory and digestive disorders related to the increased pressure put on internal organs. Also hip, knee, shoulder and neck pain, and joint dysfunction are related to abnormal forces going through our skeleton. You can appreciate why our posture is so important to our health and well-being.

There are plenty of experts out there who would love to help you fix your posture. However, if you followed what they prescribed, you would be trying to imitate their idea of what constitutes "good posture" and superimposing their idea of what that looks like. You will spend way too much time and energy focusing on what you think you *should* do, instead of what you *could* do. Once again, your posture will be stiff and rigid, without the effortless flow of neutral posture.

The following movement lessons are designed to help you find the natural curves of your spine, decrease unnecessary muscle tension, and properly align your skeletal structure. Before you begin, however, I am compelled to remind you about the fundamental principles of the *Forever Fit and Flexible* program. No matter how enthusiastic and excited you may be to get started, I encourage you to stop and review the basic principles once again before you proceed. Put the emphasis on fun, take your time, go slow, and remember that less is more.

Key Points:
- ❧ Posture is dynamic and fluid, not static and rigid.
- ❧ Everyone's posture is different according to his or her own individual structure.
- ❧ When your structure supports you, you move more easily without stress and strain.

Checkpoints:
- ❧ Move slowly and with mindful awareness.
- ❧ Focus more on what you feel rather than how you look.

Bonus Points:
- ❧ You will look taller, longer, and leaner.
- ❧ You will develop a new sense of ease, grace, and youthfulness in your posture and your carriage.

Posture Movement Lessons

Movement Lesson #1 is based on the principles of Feldenkrais and is intended to help you find the natural curves of your spine by first finding your base of support—your pelvis. Movement Lesson #2 is a combination of the principles of Feldenkrais and Pilates to gently stretch your thoracic spine and open up the front of your chest. Movement Lesson #3 is based on traditional physical therapy exercises to strengthen the muscles of the upper back as well as the shoulder blades.

Movement Lesson #1:

1. **Sit on the edge of a firm chair with your feet flat on the floor.**

   ❧ Bring your attention to your sit bones (located under each buttock and called the ischial tuberosities). Notice how your sit bones contact the chair. Take a few moments to really settle into the pressure of your sit bones against the chair.

   ❧ Notice the shape of your spine, but do not change it, fix it, move it, or make a judgment about it. Simply take the time to sense the shape of your spine from the base of your pelvis to the top of your head. Stop, sit back against your chair, and rest for a few moments.

2. **Sit on the edge of your chair with your feet flat on the floor.**

   ❧ Very slowly and gently begin to rock your pelvis forward and backward on the chair. Move from your pelvis, not from your chest. Make the movement very small, and think about moving from your skeleton instead of pushing with your muscles. Pause for a few moments. Then continue to slowly rock your pelvis for another thirty to sixty seconds. Stop. Notice how your sit bones contact the chair now. Pause for a moment.

   ❧ Begin to slowly rock your pelvis forward and backward on your sit bones. Do this several times, going even more slowly and allowing for a few moments of stillness between each repetition. Notice how the pressure of your sit bones changes against your chair as you rock your pelvis. Stop. Sit back against your chair and rest.

3. **Sit on the edge of your chair with your feet flat on the floor.**

ॐ Once again, begin rocking your pelvis forward and backward. Notice when your sit bones pass through a spot where you are balanced on your sit bones and you can comfortably sit for a minute or two. If you can sit without any effort, your spine is supporting you. You have found effortless posture in sitting.

4. **Stand up slowly.**

ॐ Notice the shape of your spine in the standing position. Walk around the room. Notice the carriage of your head, the movement of your shoulders, and the movement of your pelvis as you walk. These things may now feel different from your typical pattern of standing and walking.

Extra Credit:

ॐ Practice this movement several times during the day for maximum benefit, and as a gentle and effective way to stretch your spine and improve your posture.

Movement Lesson #2:

1. **Take a large bath towel and roll it lengthwise. Lie on the floor on your back. Bend your knees, and place your feet flat on the floor a comfortable distance apart. Place the rolled towel lengthwise under your spine and the back of your head.**

ॐ Make sure that your head is well supported and in line with your spine. You may need an additional pad placed under your head for comfort.

ॐ Take a few moments to breathe and relax on the towel roll. Gently allow your weight to sink into the roll. Slowly bring both arms over your head and toward the floor in a gentle stretch. You may need to bend your elbows to make this easier. It's important to stay within a comfortable range rather than try to force a stretch; this will be a reference point to return to later in the movement exploration. Make a mental note of how far your arms can go without straining. Notice where you might feel tight or restricted. Often, one side will be tighter than the other. Bring your arms down to your sides and rest.

ॐ Rotate your arms so that the palms of both hands are facing your thighs. Very slowly bring one arm up over your head toward the floor. Your arm does not need to be straight; instead, allow your elbow to bend. Leave your other arm down at your side. Slowly change the position of your arms, so that the bottom arm goes over your head as the top arm comes down at the same time. Make a slow scissoring motion with your arms. Slowly continue to scissor your arms with the palms facing each other. Stop and rest.

2. **Remain lying on the floor as above, with the rolled towel lengthwise under your spine and the back of your head.**

ॐ Make sure that your head is well supported and in line with your spine. You may need an additional pad under your head for comfort. Bring both arms out to your sides with your palms facing the ceiling, as if you are making the shape of a "T."

ॐ Bring one arm up over your head with the back of your hand resting on the floor, and the other arm down, next to your leg with the back of your hand resting on the floor. Slowly switch the position of your arms by sweeping the back of your hands along the floor. Continue to slowly sweep your arms like the hands of a clock with your palms facing the ceiling. Stop and rest.

3. **Remain lying on the floor as above, with the rolled towel lengthwise under your spine and the back of your head.**

   ∾ Combine the two movements together, in a "scissor-scissor-sweep" configuration.

   ∾ Start with one arm over your head and the other one down at your side with your palms facing toward your body. Slowly begin to scissor your arms. Scissor once, scissor twice, and then sweep around. As you scissor your arms, the palms face each other. As you sweep your arms, they face the ceiling. Scissor, scissor, sweep around. Continue to slowly scissor and sweep your arms. Stop and rest.

   ∾ Bring both arms over your head toward the floor and notice how far your arms can easily go without straining now. Magic, isn't it?

Movement Lesson #3:

1. **Sit on the edge of a firm chair with your feet flat on the floor.**

   ∾ Bring your elbows in close to your waistline with the palms of your hands rotating upward toward the ceiling. Slowly and firmly press your elbows *down* to the floor. Keep your head up with your eyes looking at the horizon in front of you. Hold for a few seconds.

Relax for a moment. Repeat several times. Stop and rest.

ઢ Bring your elbows in close to your waistline and the palms of your hands toward the ceiling. As you press your elbows down to the floor, imagine that the crown of your head is lengthening *up* toward the ceiling. Don't force it; just try to feel your spine getting longer as your elbows press down. Hold for a few seconds. Relax for a moment. Repeat several times. Stop and rest.

NOTE: This simple but powerful exercise can be done while standing or even when walking.

Extra Credit:

ઢ Use a foam roller instead of a towel roll to get more of a stretch through the front of your shoulders and more extension through the middle of your spine. Foam rollers can be purchased at most sporting goods stores or any other store that sells fitness equipment. Add light hand weights (start with one to two pounds) to your arm work for additional benefit. If one to two pounds feels like a little too much weight to begin with, you can start by using six-ounce tomato paste cans and progress from there.

ઢ Get more bang for your buck by standing and walking with a book on top of your head. No, I am not kidding. Models and charm schools have done this for years because it works. It is one of the oldest tricks in the book, so to speak.

chapter seven

Core Strength

*"You're more than your core,
but it sure helps to have one."*

Core strength is an important building block in your *Forever Fit and Flexible* program. Your abdominal muscles are a major component of your core strength, but core strength is more complex than merely strengthening your abdominals. Right about now, I can imagine you looking at your lower abdominals and thinking about all of the crunches and sit-ups you have tried along the way and wondering why they might not have worked out so well for you. Maybe you wrenched your neck and back in the past from trying to strengthen your core. Perhaps you are even wondering if you really have any muscles in there.

Trust me, you do, and the surprising news is that there is a fairly easy way to find your abdominal muscles and strengthen your core. Even more surprising is that you do not have to grind out sit-ups or crunches that strain your neck, hurt your back, and do nothing to target your core muscles. Are you intrigued? Allow me to shed a little light (and hope) on the subject of core strength.

Before we discuss *how* to develop core strength, we will first address *why* we need core strength. Strong core muscles support your spine and your pelvis, providing you with a stable base of support from which to move. A strong core will eliminate back pain, prevent back pain and back injuries, reinforce healthy posture, and reduce stress on your hips, knees, neck, and shoulders. Consequently, a weak core results in a protruding abdominal wall, which puts extra stress and strain on your low back. Weak core muscles also contribute to faulty posture and poor structural alignment.

I have worked with dozens of clients over the years who suffered from incapacitating chronic lower back pain and were told (by the experts) that they would just have to learn to live with it and manage the pain with rest and medication. After only a few sessions that focused on learning how to properly strengthen their core muscles, they were able to completely alleviate their back pain and return to their full level of function and activities. I clearly remember being in that exact same situation myself. Even though I was physically active, I had no idea how to effectively use my core muscles, which resulted in abnormal forces of gravity going through my spine. These forces were not the healthy forces that are necessary for a strong spine, but destructive forces that caused damage to my spine and a devastating back injury. My core muscles simply could not support my spine, and my spine collapsed under the strain.

Once I learned how to isolate and activate the proper muscles, my back pain was gone. This should be enough to persuade you to work on developing your core strength. In case you need a bit more encouragement, remember what I already mentioned—a stronger core gives you a smaller waistline. Have I captured your attention? Then keep reading.

Often when we think of strong abdominals or a strong core, we think of the six-pack or washboard abs that we see advertised in fitness magazines. The muscle that is responsible for creating the six-pack is called the rectus abdominis. The individual fibers of this muscle go up and down the front of your torso, from the lower border of the ribs to the base of the pubic bone. This means that when the muscle contracts, the fibers shorten toward each other. This action bends your spine forward and pushes your soft tissue outward, which can inadvertently develop a strong muscle that protrudes *out* rather than *in*. So, instead of being rewarded with a strong, flat belly that protects your lower back and supports your abdominal wall, you are stuck with a bigger belly that can actually place more pressure on your back and vertebral discs. To make matters even worse, all that effort expended to pump out those crunches and sit-ups can cause significant injury to your neck and back.

There is a much better, easier, and more reliable way to develop a stronger core and a flatter tummy. It is by isolating and activating an abdominal muscle that lies deep in the abdomen, called the transverse abdominis. While the fibers of the rectus abdominis go up and down, the fibers of the transverse abdominis go from side to side across the front of your torso, from the lower ribs to the pubic bone. When the muscle fibers contract, they shorten toward each other to flatten your stomach, support your internal organs, lengthen your spine, stabilize your pelvis, and protect your low back. The muscle fibers of your transverse abdominis wrap around the sides of your torso and attach to the connective tissue of your back.

This circular, multidimensional structure is what gives strong support to your low back as well as a more well-defined waistline and flatter stomach. In the Pilates community, we frequently refer to this abdominal muscle as our "girdle of strength," and my ballet master always referred to the transverse abdominis by telling us to find our "internal corset." Indeed, once you are able to find and strengthen your transverse abdominis, it does feel like you have a strong but flexible internal corset supporting you.

Let me share another fascinating bit of information with you, since we have already considered the subject of posture. This is where things start to get really interesting. When you have correct postural alignment, your spine is in the neutral position and your transverse abdominis naturally engages on its own. When you add the ability to isolate and activate your transverse abdominis, you reinforce the effortless, elegant posture that you discovered in the previous chapter. The two work together in perfect harmony.

Learning how to isolate and activate your transverse abdominis does require practice; however, once you learn how to engage this muscle, you can practice strengthening it anytime, anywhere, and in any position.

Key Points:
- A strong core helps to prevent back pain and injuries.
- You do not have to do crunches and sit-ups to strengthen your core.

Checkpoints:

- ✥ When you activate your transverse abdominis, you should only feel tension in your lower abdominals, not in your back, hips, neck, or shoulders.
- ✥ Your spine should get longer, not shorter, with the movement.

Bonus Points:

- ✥ Practice activating your transverse abdominis several times during the day to gain even more strength, stamina, and endurance of your core muscles.
- ✥ Work your transverse abdominis in the car every time you sit at a red light. It makes sitting in traffic a lot more productive, and a little bit less frustrating.

CORE STRENGTH MOVEMENT LESSONS

The following movement lessons are based on the Pilates principle of centering and will also help you discover the principle of movement flowing out from a strong center.

Movement Lesson #1:

1. **Lie down on the floor on your back. Bend your knees and place your feet flat on the floor about hip-width apart. You may need a small pad under your head for comfort.**
- ✥ Bring your attention to the shape of your low back. It should have a slight natural curve so that you can easily place your hand underneath it. Release any unnecessary tension in your low back, hips, or pelvis. Your neck should be long, with your chin slightly lifted and your eyes looking softly toward the ceiling.

- ❧ Breathe in and notice how your lower abdomen gently pooches out. When you breathe out, notice how your lower abdomen gently returns to its resting position. Take a few moments to follow the rhythm of your breathing and the natural rise and fall of your lower abdomen as you breathe.

- ❧ Bring your attention to the area in your abdomen halfway between your pubic bone and your belly button. Breathe in, let your belly gently fill and lift up as you breathe. Then, as you breathe out, gently but firmly, pull that area *in* and *up* toward your spine. Breathe in and let your belly pooch out. Breathe out and pull your lower abdominals in and up. Repeat several times and then stop and rest.

  NOTE: It is very tempting to work really hard to isolate your lower abdominals and bring everything that you have into it, including the kitchen sink. That will not benefit you; it is actually counterproductive and will sabotage your efforts to isolate and strengthen your transverse abdominis. Keep these additional checkpoints in mind while you go through the process of re-training your abdominal muscles.

- ❧ The shape of your back, pelvis, and neck against the floor does not change as you contract your lower abdominals.

- ❧ Be careful not to flatten your low back or the back of your neck into the floor.

- ❧ Keep your jaw relaxed and your face and eyes soft.

- ❧ You should still have no tension in your low back, hips, or pelvis.

- ❧ The only area where you should feel tension is deep in your lower abdominals.

2. **Take a few moments to imagine the shape of your transverse abdominis.**

   ❧ Imagine the fibers of that muscle going across the front of your torso from right to left. Think about how the fibers come together to flatten your abdomen and lengthen your spine as they shorten (contract).

   ❧ Focus on the rise and fall of your breathing. Pull your lower abdominals in with each exhale, keeping the shape of your transverse abdominis in your attention as you do the movement. Imagine that the fibers of the transverse abdominis are firmly but gently pulling in your lower belly. Slowly repeat this several times, then stop and rest.

   ❧ Once again, focus on your breathing and pull your lower abdominals in with each exhale, activating your transverse abdominis. This time, keep your transverse abdominis firmly engaged while you breathe in and out; you are actually doing an isometric contraction of your transverse abdominis. Keep the lower abdominals taut and your neck, jaw, face, hips, and low back relaxed while you isolate the abdominals. Continue for thirty to sixty seconds, then stop and rest. Repeat three to five times. Stop.

Movement Lesson #2:

1. **Sit on the edge of a firm chair with your feet flat on the floor.**

   ❧ Take a moment to find the neutral position of your spine and pelvis while sitting, just as you did in the chapter on posture.

   ❧ Breathe in and let your lower belly protrude out slightly. Breathe out and firmly pull your lower belly in, without changing the shape of your low back or pelvis. Breathe in and release your abdominals. Slowly and thoughtfully repeat the movement several times until you can feel your lower abdominals working. Stop and rest for a moment.

NOTE: You are simply repeating Movement Lesson #1, but in a sitting position.

ॐ Take a few moments to imagine the shape of your transverse abdominis. Visualize the fibers of that muscle going across your torso from right to left. Once again, follow the rhythm of your breathing. Firmly and gently pull your lower abdominals in with each exhale. You should get a bit taller as you tighten your lower abs. There should be no tension in your hips, legs, chest, neck, or shoulders. Stop and rest.

2. **Sit on the edge of your chair with your feet flat on the floor.**

ॐ Once again, follow the rhythm of your breathing and firmly pull your lower belly in when you exhale, activating your transverse abdominis. Keep your transverse abdominis firmly engaged while you breathe in and out instead of allowing it to pooch out when you breathe in. Remember to lengthen your spine as you pull in your transverse abdominis. Continue to keep the lower abdominals taut as you breathe for thirty to sixty seconds, then stop and rest. Repeat three to five times. Stop.

ॐ Repeat the above step, noticing how long you can keep the tension low in your abdominals without causing any tension in your hips, back, chest, neck, and shoulders. Lengthen your spine. Stop and rest.

☙ Stand up. Pay attention to the length of your spine, the carriage of your head, and the gentle tension in your lower abdominals. Practice the gentle contraction of your lower abdominals up and in toward the front of your spine while standing, without changing the shape of your back.

NOTE: Not only are you strengthening your core muscles with this series of movements, you are also finding something that we in the Pilates community refer to as "axial elongation." It is a way of lengthening your spine all the way from the tailbone to the cranium, and helps you further improve your posture.

Extra Credit:

☙ Invest in a series of private Pilates sessions with a qualified and experienced instructor. I highly recommend beginning with the Pilates Reformer, which provides support and gentle assistance to help you isolate and strengthen your core. However, if you do have neck or back pain or recent injuries, are recovering from surgery, or are significantly overweight or out of shape, look for a Pilates instructor who also has a background in physical therapy. Once you develop a stronger core and a better sense of body awareness and control, you can progress to small group classes. To further challenge yourself and advance your core strengthening, have your instructor teach you the original mat exercises created by Joseph Pilates. Just a few minutes a day at home on the floor can help you rapidly and effectively improve your core strength as well as your posture and flexibility.

chapter eight

Flexibility

"If you can't bend your knees,
you can't do squat."

Most of us experience a loss of flexibility as we get older and we seem to accept it as a "normal" part of the aging process. However, our activity level (or lack thereof) has a much greater impact on our flexibility than getting older does.

I still have a vivid memory from one of my textbooks when I was in physical therapy school. It was a chart comparing the degenerative effects of injuries, a sedentary lifestyle, and the aging process on human tissues and flexibility. Guess what the chart showed? The least destructive impact on flexibility was the "aging process," while the most detrimental effect was a consequence of a sedentary lifestyle. I guess that explains why that beautiful woman rehearsing her dance routine was able to effortlessly get up from her chair by doing a fan kick with her legs. It also validates my humble opinion that sitting is evil and why it took me so long to regain my flexibility after graduate school. So, take heart; we don't have to lose flexibility as we mature. However, even if we are physically active and stretch our muscles on a regular basis, we can still feel stiff and tight. That's because, contrary to popular belief, improving our flexibility is not as simple as just trying to stretch tight muscles.

Often, a loss of flexibility is not a direct result of tight muscles, but arises from a lack of mobility in our joints. This loss of movement in our joints causes a shortening and tightening of the connective tissue surrounding the joints along with a sensation of tightness in our muscles. Prolonged sitting, standing, forward posture, working at a computer, or a sedentary lifestyle can leave you stuck in this position and screaming for relief from the Tin Man's oil can. Remember my disastrous return to ballet class after sitting in physical therapy school twelve hours a day, seven days a week, for two years? Even if you are physically active, repetitive motion, faulty movement patterns, or holding certain positions for an extended period of time can lead to a downhill spiral of joint dysfunction and loss of flexibility.

Our joints have a wide range of motion that is naturally available to them. If we don't use our joints to their full capacity, the soft tissue surrounding the joints shortens and contracts, pulling on our muscles and joints. As the soft tissue gets tighter, we lose the ability to move our joints, and our range of motion decreases. As a result, the tissues continue to get tighter, and then we lose even more range of motion.

A vicious cycle has begun. It is a classic example of use

it or lose it, or more accurately, *move it* or lose it. We usually do not recognize the insidious onset of loss of joint function and mobility, but it does capture our attention when we start to feel tight and stiff. We might try traditional stretching techniques, thinking that these efforts will help us loosen up and improve our flexibility. Think again. The following explanation is what happens when we try and stretch tight muscles without first addressing our joint mobility.

Our muscles are inherently elastic, and have a rich blood supply to help keep them that way. However, where muscles attach to the bones and joints, the tissue changes into much less elastic tissue in the form of tendons, ligaments, and other connective tissue. These tissues have very little blood supply, but they do have an abundance of nerve fibers that are responsible for protecting our joints. When we try to stretch tight muscles in a direction in which our joint is already compromised, the nerve fibers get the message that our joint is in danger of being injured. These fibers then transmit warning signals to our brain, which in turn send the message back to our muscles to tighten up even further to protect the joint. The muscles become tighter than they were before we stretched, and our joint mobility is even further compromised.

The good news is that we can improve our flexibility by first lubricating our joints with gentle movement and joint mobilization. This relaxes and loosens the soft tissues surrounding our joints, stimulates healthy joint function, and gets the synovial fluid moving in our joints. Synovial fluid is a viscous substance that helps lubricate our joints and functions as our own internal oil can. Once we get our joints moving more easily and more naturally, we can get a lot more benefit from stretching our muscles.

Key Points:

- ❧ Traditional stretches will not improve your flexibility unless accompanied with gentle joint mobility.
- ❧ Improving your flexibility will help improve your posture.

Checkpoints:

- ❧ Remember to make very small movements.
- ❧ Work within a comfortable range of motion without strain or discomfort. Do not try to reach your limits or your end range of motion.

Bonus Points:

- ❧ Practice getting up and down from the floor. This simple act is a powerful tool to improve your flexibility, as well as your balance and strength.

FLEXIBILITY MOVEMENT LESSONS

The following movement lessons are based on The Feldenkrais Method® and the principle that gentle movement of our joints through an easy range of motion allows our nervous system to relax the soft tissue supporting them.

Movement Lesson #1:

1. **Stand with your feet about hip-width apart and your arms at your side.**
   - ❧ Take some time to notice the shape of your low back and the curves of your spine. Notice if your back feels tight and stiff, or soft and relaxed.
   - ❧ Relax your knees so that they bend slightly. Stay like that for a moment and notice the shape and sensa-

tions of your low back in this position. Straighten your knees as much as you can and notice how, once again, the shape and sensations in your low back change. Slowly go back and forth between keeping your knees softly bent or very straight, paying close attention to the shape and feelings in your low back. Stop and rest in a sitting position, or walk around the room for a moment.

2. Come back to your standing position.

ক Slowly go back and forth from slightly and gently bending your knees to then straightening them. Move slowly and gently through a very small range of motion. This time, pay attention to the changing of the shape and the sensations in your hips, knees, and ankles. If you feel any sense of discomfort, make the movement even smaller. Stop and pause for a few moments.

ক Slowly return to slightly bending and then straightening your knees, with your attention on your hips, knees, and ankles. You may even begin to notice an increase in the range of motion in these joints, or an ease in the quality of movement. Stop and then walk around the room.

3. Come back to your standing position.

ক Slightly bend your knees. Now, with your knees slightly bent, slowly shift your weight side to side. Go very slowly, make the movement smooth and continuous, and pay attention to the movement in your hips joints. Stop and walk around the room.

ক Stop walking and stand with your knees slightly bent.

Begin to make small, slow, easy circles with your hips and pelvis. Feel how one knee bends a bit more than the other as you circle in one direction and how that changes as you circle the other way. Each time you circle your pelvis, notice how the movement becomes easier and more fluid. Stop, walk around the room for a few minutes, and notice the difference in how you walk, as well as the sensations in your back, hips, knees, and ankles.

NOTE: We have a saying in my martial arts training "let your knees be your teacher." This movement lesson in softening your knees by slightly bending them can decrease tension in your low back, help you feel more grounded, and improve your balance as well as your flexibility. Make sure that you bend your knees *slightly* and do not go into a mini-squat. That comes later with strengthening.

Movement Lesson #2:

1. **Get down on the floor onto your hands and knees. You may need to place a small pad under your knees for comfort.**

   - Make sure that your shoulders are directly over your hands and your hips are directly over your knees. Allow your neck to relax so that your head lowers down slightly and your eyes gently look toward the floor.
   - Slowly begin to shift your weight forward over your hands. Slowly return back to your starting position. Then shift your weight backward so that your tailbone goes back toward your heels. Start with a very small range of motion and gradually increase the range in small increments as the movement gets easier and more comfortable. Stop and rest in any position.

2. **Return to your hands and knees. Keep your neck relaxed and your eyes looking toward the floor.**

ও Allow the area between your shoulder blades to sink down a bit, as if your breastbone is gently yielding to gravity toward the floor. Then firmly push your hands against the floor to return to your starting position. Make the movement very small and very slow, as you lower and lift the area between your shoulder blades. Continue to play with this movement and notice how your pelvis and your head respond to this movement. Stop and rest in any position.

3. **Return to your hands and knees. Keep your neck relaxed and your eyes looking toward the floor.**

ও Begin to do the same movement, lowering and lifting the area between your shoulder blades.

ও Notice that when the area between your shoulder blades sinks down, your pelvis and tailbone naturally lift toward the ceiling and your head gently lifts up. As the area between your shoulder blades lifts up, your pelvis, tailbone, and head lower toward the floor. Take the time to enjoy this total body experience. Then, stop and rest in any position.

4. **Return to your hands and knees. Keep your neck relaxed and your eyes looking toward the floor.**

ও Begin to do the same movement, lowering and lifting the area between your shoulder blades.

ও When your shoulder blades sink down and your tailbone and head lift up, let your belly expand out. When you push your hands against the floor, firmly pull your lower abdominals in, and hold it for a few seconds. You are adding both the component of pelvic rocking that you learned in Chapter Five with the element of core strengthening that you learned in Chapter Six. Do you notice how it all comes together? How cool is that?

Movement Lesson #3:

1. **Stand up with your feet about hip-width apart and your knees slightly bent.**

    ❧ Bring your right arm up in front of you, straight out from your shoulder, as if you are pointing at something. Keep your eyes focused on your right hand as you slowly and gently move your arm and simultaneously turn your head and eyes to the right, as if you are going to point at something behind you. Move only as far as you can comfortably go without straining or stretching. Make a mental note of how far you have moved by locating a spot on the wall or other landmark behind you. Bring your arm and head back to your starting place, following your hand with your eyes, then lower your arm and rest a moment.

    ❧ Lift your right arm again in front of you and gently move your arm, along with your head and eyes, to the right, as if you are once again pointing at something behind you. Leave your arm and shoulders to the right, and then slowly and gently turn your head and eyes to the left to look over your left shoulder. Slowly bring your head and eyes to the right to look at your right arm and hand once more. Again, turn your eyes and head to look over your left shoulder, while keeping your arm and shoulders to the right. Turn again to the right. Now bring your right arm, eyes, head, and shoulders back to face front and lower your arm. Stop and rest.

- ❧ One last time, lift your right arm in front of you. Keep your eyes focused on your right hand as you slowly and gently simultaneously move your arm and turn your head and eyes to the right, as if you are again going to point at something behind you. Notice how far you can now easily perform this movement and compare this to when you first did the movement. Notice the change in your range of motion as well as the ease and the quality of your movement.

2. **Repeat #1 on the other side.**
   NOTE: This wonderful little exercise opens up the individual joints along the length of your spine and activates a reflex in your brain called the vestibular-ocular reflex. This reflex helps decrease the excess muscle tone in the neck, and also plays a pivotal role in balance.

Movement Lesson #4:

1. **Lie down on the floor on your back. Bend your knees and place your feet flat on the floor, about hip-width apart. You may need a small pad under your head for comfort.**

- ❧ Slowly lengthen your legs one at a time until both of your knees are straight. Moving one leg at a time, bend them again until both knees are bent with your feet flat on the floor.

- ❧ Slowly go back and forth between straightening your legs and bending them again. Notice the trajectory of your knees and the relationship of your knees to the ceiling as you bend and straighten your legs. Are your knees facing the ceiling as you move your legs, or are they rolling out to the side? Notice the sensation in your hips and your low back as you move. Stop and rest.

2. **Lie down on the floor on your back. Bend your knees and place your feet flat on the floor, about hip-width apart.**

ॐ Keep your left leg in the bent knee position. Slowly allow your right knee to open out to the side and then slowly lengthen your leg against the floor until your right leg is straight in a slightly rotated-out position with your baby toe resting on the floor. Pause for a moment. Keeping your baby toe against the floor, bend your knee and begin to slide your right foot toward your buttocks. Your right leg is still in contact with the floor. Now, bring your right knee toward the ceiling so that you are back to your starting position with both knees bent and feet flat on the floor. Repeat this movement several times. Stop and rest. **NOTE:** The trajectory of your knee is crucial to this movement lesson. As your knee rolls outward (in a position of external rotation), your hip joint is allowed to gently and naturally roll, slide, and glide in the socket allowing for more range of motion and flexibility in your hip. This will also decrease stress and strain on your low back (lumbar spine). As a test, try several times to bend and straighten your right leg by keeping the path of your knee directly toward the ceiling and notice the sensations and range of motion in your hip joint. Pause for a moment. Now bend and straighten your knee by keeping the path of your knee oriented toward the wall rather than the ceiling. Notice the sensations and range of motion in your hip now. Often we use our hip joints as a hinge joint, moving forward and backward instead of performing the circular, multi-dimensional movement they were designed to perform.

৯ Keep your right leg in the bent knee position. Slowly allow your left knee to open out to the side and then slowly lengthen your leg against the floor until your left leg is straight in a slightly rotated-out position with your baby toe resting on the floor. Pause for a moment. Keeping your baby toe against the floor, bend your knee and begin to slide your left foot toward your buttocks. Your left leg is still in contact with the floor. Now, bring your left knee toward the ceiling so that you are back to your starting position with both knees bent and feet flat on the floor. Repeat this movement several times. Stop and rest.

3. **Lie down on the floor on your back. Bend your knees and place your feet flat on the floor, about hip-width apart.**

৯ Slowly let your right knee roll out to the side and slide your right foot against the floor until your leg is straight and baby toe is resting against the floor. Slowly let your left knee roll out to the side and slide your left foot against the floor so that both legs are straight and rotated outward. Pause for a moment. Now reverse the process. Keeping your baby toe against the floor, bend your right knee and begin to slide your right foot toward your buttocks. Your right leg is still in contact with the floor. Now, bring your right knee toward the ceiling so that you are back to your starting position with your right knee bent and right foot flat on the floor. Do the same movement with your left leg so that both knees are once again bent toward the ceiling and both feet are flat on the floor. Stop and rest.

❧ Continue to straighten and bend your alternating legs as described above for a few more repetitions, then stop and rest. As you practice this movement, allow your pelvis to roll with the movement of your legs. Notice the trajectory of your knees and the relationship of your knees to the ceiling as you bend and straighten your legs. Notice the sensation in your hips and your low back as you move. Stop and rest.

Extra Credit:

❧ There are so many different activities and modalities that can help you improve your flexibility and joint range of motion. Of course, I have already addressed four of them in Chapter 3. These include Pilates, Feldenkrais, dance, and martial arts. All of these are fantastic methods to improve your flexibility. They will also increase your body awareness, posture, core, balance, strength, and fitness at the same time. But, what I really love most about all of these movement arts is that you will learn movement patterns and exercises that you can do at home on your own. I suggest that you do your homework, research what is available in your area, and check out some classes. It will be well worth your time and effort.

chapter nine

Balance

"Don't let the rug get pulled
out from underneath you."

Balance is another vital component to our fitness and flex-ibility. Most of the time, we think that good balance is simply the ability to stand up without falling over. But it is much more complex than that. Balance refers to our ability to make adjustments within ourselves to adapt to our environ-ment when it abruptly and unexpectedly changes, such as walking on uneven surfaces, changes in terrain, or standing on a moving platform.

A lot of us are afraid of falling, especially as we get older. As babies and small children, we lived, played, and crawled on the floor. As we grew, we continued to frequently get down on the floor. The occasional spills we experienced were no big deal, and we would bounce back up and be off on our next adventure. Granted, we were also much shorter and closer to the ground, so we did not have as far to fall. We also spent a lot of our playtime on the floor, so being on the floor was familiar territory to us. Not so much as we get older.

As adults, we keep ourselves upright. We stand, walk, sit in chairs, and lose our intimate relationship with the ground. As a result, we develop a fear and distrust of the ground, of our ability to fall safely (yes, there is such a thing) and gracefully get back up. Since we spend a lot less time on the floor, it gets more difficult to get up and down from the floor.

Being on the floor is now unfamiliar territory to us and even just thinking about it makes us uncomfortable, doesn't it? This can further develop into a fear of falling, decreasing flexibility and declining balance. But fear not—the floor is our friend, and it is a powerful teacher that can help us improve our balance.

An interesting technique to improve our balance is to practice falling. No, I'm not kidding, although I will admit that it is easier said than done. I don't advise doing it, though, unless you are in a safe and controlled environment with someone instructing you. Alternatively, there are movements you can begin to do by yourself. You can start by simply getting down on the floor every day to practice rolling around and getting back up. It might sound silly, but it's a very effective method to help your balance as well as keep you *fit and flexible*.

One of my clients, Betty, had terrible balance when she first came to me for Pilates conditioning. Her balance, strength, and flexibility were so compromised that she couldn't get on and off the reformer without my help, let alone get on the floor. After a few months, Betty progressively needed less assistance until the time came when she was able to maneuver around and get on and off the equipment without any help at all. Remarkably, her balance dramatically improved as well, which absolutely delighted her.

However, her ability to get down on the floor was another story. Not only did she need help getting to the floor, she couldn't stay there for very long before pain began to shoot across her back and her knees. Since Pilates had worked so well for her, Betty decided to sign up for a series of Feldenkrais classes, even though they were going to be done lying on the floor in typical Feldenkrais fashion.

The first class didn't work very well for her, and I could tell she was experiencing a lot of discomfort. I gave her several suggestions for changing her position or even doing the lesson sitting in a chair, but she pushed through the lesson while lying on her back. She ended up with back pain for the next few days but showed up for the second class the following week. Her back was still a little sore, so this time she decided to do the lesson sitting in a chair to see if that helped. It did, but she had back pain again after the class.

By the time the third class in the series came along, Betty was *still* experiencing low back pain. I was ready to give her a full refund for the entire series, but something extraordinary happened during that last class. Her body began to change and integrate the movements from the two previous classes. Betty looked a lot more comfortable, and she moved in an easy and effortless manner. Although she did the lesson sitting in the chair, she used her imagination to "see" herself doing the lesson lying on the floor. Most amazing, her back didn't hurt at all after that class. At the end of every class, I give my clients one simple tip that they can take home and practice. After this third class, I recommended that everyone get down on the floor at least once a day. I did get a few skeptical looks, but because I am truly passionate about the powerful benefits of getting on the floor, I knew it would benefit each and every participant. As I said, the floor is our friend.

The following week when Betty came to her Pilates workout, she told me she thought about my tip but wasn't able to get on the floor. She just couldn't do it. "Well, then, don't worry about it," I told her. "You're doing great and you have made so much progress. Take some time to enjoy your success." About a month later, the magic happened. During Pilates, Betty casually mentioned that she was getting on the floor every day just like I suggested. Not just once a day, but twice, each and every day. I was flabbergasted. She told me that she had continued to work on it until she figured out how to do it. She actually told me that my recommendation to get on the floor each day was the best tip she'd ever received, and she was amazed by how much better her balance was from that simple tip. The most exciting part of this story is that she is expecting her first grandchild soon, and Grannie is going to be able to crawl around on the floor with her grandbaby. Go, Grannie, go!

Another longtime client and friend was thinking about moving her laundry room from her basement to the main floor of her ranch-style home so she and her husband wouldn't have to climb the stairs as often. When she heard my tip about the floor, she had one of those head-smacking moments. She realized that if she didn't *have* to climb the stairs, then she *wouldn't* climb the stairs, and it was just a matter of time before she *couldn't* manage the stairs. She knew that would have a serious impact on her balance and mobility, as well as increase her risk of falling as she got older. Clever lady! Her laundry room remains in the basement, exactly where it was for years.

The first thing I learned when I began studying martial arts was how to fall. It would be more accurate to say I learned how to land without getting hurt. I have always hated the thought of falling, and as a dancer I worked very hard to stay in the upright position. Even on the ski slopes, I was always cautious and careful not to end up in a snow bank. My father, who was an excellent skier as well as a martial artist, would tease me mercilessly for being so afraid to fall. Easy for him to say; he never fell down. Well, hardly ever.

I'll never forget the time my husband and I were skiing with him and my sister. My father hit a rock and went flying down the slope out of control. It was a spectacular fall, and my husband quickly skied down to see if he was okay. By the time my sister and I got to him, my dad was still on the ground, and I thought we were going to have to call the ski patrol. Then I noticed why he wasn't getting up; he was rolling around in the snow and roaring with laughter. I guessed he wasn't hurt. My husband exclaimed, "Wow, George! That was a really impressive fall! You fell like a thirty-year-old!" Still laughing, my father finally got up and replied, "Yes, but I got up like a forty-year-old!" He was in his mid-sixties at the time. Almost twenty years later, he tripped over a tree root in his yard, and once again, went flying down another steep hill. He was not hurt and later told us that he instinctively and reflexively tucked into a karate roll. My father sure knew how to fall, and he also knew how to get back up.

A few years ago my husband and I were hiking and ended up on a trail that was covered with snow and ice. It was a holiday weekend, so the trail was packed with hikers, most of them completely unprepared for the conditions. We were only halfway up the trail when I started to worry about the trip down. We were okay going up, but the trip down was going to be an entirely different story. I suspected it would be downright treacherous. I knew I would have to figure out a strategy to get back down in one piece. Once we started our descent, not only did we have to deal with the hazardous conditions, we had to maneuver around the other hikers trying to make their way down the trail. It was fascinating to watch how some of the hikers were choosing to get down the mountain.

One group of teenagers took a running start and then slid down the glaciers as if they were skiing on their sneakers. An interesting technique, considering the huge rocks, large trees, sharp drops into the canyon, as well as the fact that a few of them were carrying large, pointed sticks for balance. I envisioned a few trips to the local emergency room.

One woman walked behind her husband with her arms wrapped around his waist for security. This put her in a position where she was bent forward with her center of gravity in front of her base of support, not a good place to be under the best of circumstances, let alone on that mountain. She fell twice, once with her husband hanging on to her arm. As I watched, I was actually more concerned that he would dislocate her shoulder trying to keep her from falling than if he just let her fall, or at least guided her to the ground rather than yanking on her arm. Another family had two small girls who looked terrified as their dad tied a rope around their waists and then around his own. Yikes! I couldn't bear to think about what would happen if he fell, taking his little girls with him.

Without even thinking, I set my weight down into my pelvis, lowered my center of gravity directly over my base of support, kept my upper body flexible, and shifted my weight side to side. I quickly and confidently scampered down the mountain. Even if I did fall, I intuitively knew that I wouldn't get hurt. My center of gravity was so low and close to the ground that I didn't have far to fall.

Of course, I had the advantage of having studied a martial art where we learned how to lower our center of gravity and how to move in a manner that helps us stay connected to the ground while we glide over it. I'm going to share a few of these secrets with you in the movement lessons at the end of this chapter.

Balance is not about being able to remain upright by holding ourselves rigid and inflexible; it is about keeping our center of gravity over our base of support and allowing for movement to flow through us. Balance is also about being able to maintain our equilibrium under any circumstances. Just as we have nerve fibers that help protect our joints by responding to stretch, we have nerve fibers that respond to our position and our relationship to our environment. These nerve fibers (receptors) exist throughout our body as well as within our inner ear canal to help us maintain our equilibrium. Our feet, ankles, and hips especially have a tremendous amount of these nerve endings.

These nerve receptors transmit signals to our brain to help us correct our position in space when we lose our footing. As we mature, they do not fire as quickly as when we were younger, especially if we do not challenge them by capturing their attention. It is another example of use it or lose it. The good news is that you have already begun to fine-tune the awareness of your balance receptors by improving your posture, core strength, and flexibility. That is a fantastic start, and now it is time to take it a few steps further.

Key Points:
- ❧ Balance involves making adjustments to our environment, not holding our body still or rigid.
- ❧ The floor is a powerful teacher to help us improve our balance.

Checkpoints:
- ❧ Hold onto a countertop or other stable surface for safety.
- ❧ Allow for wobbling in your hips and ankles as you practice your standing balance. This is an important part of balance training.

Bonus Points:
- ❧ Take a few minutes every day to get down on the floor and crawl around. Make friends with the floor; besides, you never know what you may discover while you're down there.

BALANCE MOVEMENT LESSONS

Movement Lessons #1 and #2 are based on traditional physical therapy balance training exercises and are intended to improve the reflexes of the nerve endings in your feet, ankles, knees, and hips. Movement Lesson #3 is based on Feldenkrais and will increase the strength, flexibility, and sensitivity of your feet as well as improve your balance. Movement Lesson #4 is founded on one of the basic principles of martial arts. It is a technique that helps you stay grounded and balanced as well as provides you with options for moving in different directions, including backward.

Movement Lesson #1:

1. **Stand with your feet about hip-width apart in front of a countertop or other stable surface.**
   - You can do this movement lesson in your bare feet or in shoes, whichever is more comfortable for you. I prefer bare feet.
   - Place your hands on the countertop for safety. Lift your right foot off the floor so that you are standing on your left leg. Do not rest your lifted foot against your standing leg. Instead, allow it to dangle in the air in a relaxed position. You can lift your hands off the counter if you feel comfortable, but to effectively improve your balance, it's not necessary. Balance on one leg for thirty to sixty seconds. Stop, lower your foot, and rest for a moment. Repeat two more times.
   - Place your hands on the countertop for safety. Lift your left foot off the floor so you are standing on your right leg. Feel free to lift your hands off the countertop if you are comfortable. Balance for thirty to sixty seconds. Stop, lower your foot, and rest for a moment. Repeat two more times.

2. **Stand with your feet about hip-width apart in front of a countertop or other stable surface.**
   - Place your hands on the countertop for safety. Lift your right foot off the floor so that you are standing on your left leg. This time slightly bend your left knee, and balance in this position for thirty to sixty seconds. (You may notice that this is a bit more challenging. You may also notice more wobbling in your hip and ankle.) Stop, lower your foot, and rest for a moment. Repeat two more times.

ـ৯ Place your hands on the countertop for safety. Lift your left foot off the floor so that you are standing on your right leg. Slightly bend your right knee and balance in this position for thirty to sixty seconds. Stop, lower your foot, and rest for a moment. Repeat two more times.

Movement Lesson #2:
1. Stand in front of the countertop as before.

ـ৯ Place a small pillow under your left foot, and lift your right foot off the floor so that you are balancing on your left leg. The pillow decreases the stability of your standing surface, providing a further challenge for your balance and an opportunity to improve it with practice. Balance for thirty to sixty seconds, using the countertop for support when you need it. Stop and rest for a moment. Repeat two more times.

ـ৯ Put the pillow under your right foot. Lift your left foot off the floor so that you are balancing on your right leg. Balance for thirty to sixty seconds. Stop and rest for a moment. Repeat two more times.

2. Stand in front of the countertop.

ـ৯ Place the small pillow under your left foot. Lift your right foot off the floor, slightly bend your left knee, and balance for thirty to sixty seconds. Stop and rest. Repeat two more times.

ـ৯ Place the pillow under your right foot. Lift your left leg off the floor, slightly bend your right knee, and balance for thirty to sixty seconds. Stop and rest for a moment. Repeat two more times.

NOTE: When it feels easy to balance on one leg with

a small pillow under your standing foot, you can further challenge yourself by adding additional pillows
to stand on.

Movement Lesson #3:

1. **Sit on the edge of a firm chair with your bare feet flat against a carpet or throw rug on the floor. This will not work on hardwood or tile.**

   - Take a moment to notice how your feet contact the floor. Briskly rub both feet back and forth by alternating your feet so that as one is sliding forward the other is sliding backward. Continue for a few seconds. Stop. Notice the sensations on the bottom of your feet, and notice how this movement pattern seems to "wake up" the bottoms of your feet. Notice how your feet contact the floor now.

   - Once again, rub your feet briskly against the floor. Continue for a few seconds. Stop. Notice the sensations in the bottoms of your feet. Stand and notice how your feet contact the floor in a standing position. Walk around the room a bit, again noticing how your feet contact the floor as well as the movement of your feet.

2. **Sit on the edge of a firm chair with both feet flat against the floor.**

   - Slowly lift and lower all the toes of your right foot while the rest of your foot remains firmly against the floor. It might take a few repetitions to isolate the movement of your toes from your foot. Don't lift any other part of your foot except your toes. Stop and rest.

ॐ Slowly lift and lower the toes of your right foot. Add the motion to spread all your toes as you lift them off the floor while keeping the rest of your foot firmly against the floor. If this is challenging for you, it will get easier with practice.

ॐ Once again, lift and spread the toes of your right foot as you keep the rest of your foot on the floor. Now slowly lower your toes down to the floor, one at a time, beginning with the baby toe and slowly working your way through all five toes. This does take some practice, but it will greatly improve the flexibility of your feet, which is essential for balance.

ॐ Repeat the above lesson with your left foot. Once this gets easier for you, you can work both feet at the same time.

3. **Sit on the edge of a firm chair with both feet flat against the floor.**

ॐ Slowly lift and lower the ball of your right foot as you keep your heel and all five toes on the floor. As the ball of your foot lifts off the floor, your toes will slide against the carpet. You are simply going in the opposite direction of the previous movement pattern. Stop and rest.

ॐ Continue lifting and lowering the ball of your right foot against the floor. Focus on each individual toe as it slides on the carpet. Notice if the movement begins to get easier with each repetition. Stop and rest.

ॐ Repeat with your left foot. You can also work both feet at the same time once you are comfortable with the movement pattern.

Movement Lesson #4:

1. **Stand in the center of a room in your stocking feet on a tile or hardwood floor.**

   ✐ Stand with your feet about hip-width apart. Gently bend your knees and slowly begin to shift your weight side to side a few times. Feel your back relax and your pelvis get a little lower to the floor. Stop for a moment and walk around the room.

   ✐ Stand with your feet about hip-width apart and your knees bent. Place your right foot slightly in front of you and slowly shift your weight forward and back. Keep your head up and focus on moving from your hips and your pelvis rather than leaning forward with your head and chest. Make sure that your right knee is going directly over the first two toes of your right foot. Stop and rest.

   ✐ Stand with your feet about hip-width apart and your knees bent. Place your left foot slightly in front of you and slowly shift your weight forward and back. Keep your head up and focus on moving from your hips and your pelvis rather than leaning forward with your head and chest. Make sure that your left knee is going directly over the first two toes of your left foot. Stop and rest.

2. **Stand in the center of a room in your stocking feet on a tile or hardwood floor.**

   ✐ Stand with your feet about hip-width apart with your knees bent. Move forward by slowly sliding your right foot forward against the floor, then slide your left foot forward to meet it. Slowly slide your left foot forward against the floor, then slide your right foot forward to meet it. Remember to keep your head up instead of looking at the floor or your feet. Continue to move forward by sliding your feet and alternating sides, as if you are skating across the floor. Stop for a moment.

≥ Stand with your feet about hip-width apart with your knees bent. Once again begin to "skate" across the floor by alternating your feet and sliding against the floor. Keep your head up and make sure that you are moving from your hips and your pelvis rather than leaning forward and leading from your head or chest. Stop for a moment.

3. **Stand in the center of a room in your stocking feet on a tile or hardwood floor.**

≥ Stand with your feet about hip-width apart. Gently place your hands in front of your belly as if you are holding a soccer ball. Leave your hands in this position, bend your knees, and once again begin to "skate" forward, focusing on your imaginary soccer ball leading the way and guiding your path forward until you cross the length of the room. Keep your head up and move from your hips and pelvis. Stop for a moment.

≥ Turn around to face the other direction. Stand with your feet hip-width apart, place your hands in front of your belly, bend your knees, and "skate" the length of the room. Continue to "skate" back and forth across the length of the floor. Remember, keep your head up and move from your hips and pelvis. Stop for a moment.

4. **Stand in the center of a room in your stocking feet on a tile or hardwood floor.**

☙ Before you start this movement pattern make sure that there are no obstacles behind you that could get in your way. Stand with your feet about hip-width apart and bend your knees. Move backward by slowly sliding your right foot backward against the floor, then slide your left foot to meet it. Slowly slide your left foot backward against the floor, then slide your right foot to meet it. Continue to move backward by sliding your feet as if you are skating across the floor. Stop for a moment.

☙ Stand with your feet about hip-width apart. Bend your knees and once again begin to "skate" backward across the floor by alternating sliding your feet against the floor. Keep your head and spine upright and in neutral alignment with your hips and pelvis. **NOTE:** Moving backward through space is a challenge, because we don't do it in our daily life. As a consequence of always propelling ourselves forward, we narrow our ability to fully sense and move through our environment. This results in further limitations in our balance, awareness, reflexes, and proprioception (the ability to sense where you are in relation to your environment). Really slow yourself down as you go through the backward movement lesson, and try to "feel" the air and the room behind you with your back. It is more important to focus on how you can become more sensitive to the space behind you than it is to complete the movement of actually going backward. Do not practice skating backward until you have accomplished the ability to sense and feel what is behind you as you slowly experience the lesson.

5. Stand in the center of a room in your stocking feet on a tile or hardwood floor.

∂ Stand with your feet about hip-width apart. Gently place your hands in front of your belly as if you are holding a soccer ball. Leave your hands in this position, bend your knees, and once again begin to "skate" backward. As you move backward focus on your mid-back and lower back leading the way and guiding your path backward until you cross the length of the room. Keep your head up. Stop for a moment.

∂ Stand with your feet hip-width apart, place your hands in front of your belly, bend your knees, and "skate" forward the length of the room. Without turning around, "skate" backward the length of the room. Play with alternating going forward and backward while you focus on moving from your hips and your pelvis as you go forward, with your mid-back and lower back leading the way as you go backward. Remember to keep your head up! Stop, walk around, and notice how your walking pattern is different than it was before you started this movement lesson.

Extra Credit:

∂ At the risk of repeating myself, Pilates, Feldenkrais, dance, and martial arts can help you further challenge and improve your balance, in addition to all the other benefits we have already talked about.

∂ Invest in an exercise ball to use at home. Just sitting and gently bouncing on a large exercise ball will help you improve your balance and proprioception. I highly recommend that you invest in a private session with a physical therapist to learn how to use the ball safely and effectively, as well as to make sure you buy the correct size for you. Once you know how to use the ball safely, you can alternate sitting on the ball when you are working on your computer, doing paperwork, or for brief intervals while watching television. Sitting and gently bouncing on the ball is a terrific way to get your circulation moving and your metabolism going. It also relieves stress and makes you feel more alert.

∽ If you really want to take it to the next level, find a supervised environment where you can safely practice falling, such as at a beginning martial arts class on a padded mat. You will learn a skill that may come in handy someday.

chapter ten

Functional Strength

"Strong is sexy, at every age."

Muscles are a must, because a strong body is a healthy body, and it is an attractive one as well. There is nothing more appealing than the look of sleek, toned muscles in every stage of life. But even more important than the way a strong body *looks* is the way it *feels*. Strength feels healthy, confident, resilient, and youthful. Strength is imperative for healthy function, but strong muscles help us in many other ways as well.

Strong muscles increase our metabolism and help us burn calories. That alone should be enough to make you want to pick up some weights and get started. But there's even more good news. Strong muscles also lead to strong bones. By putting a healthy load of stress on our muscles to build them, we also place a healthy stress on our bones at the same time. When we stress our bones, we strengthen them. It is a phenomenon called Wolf's Law, and we can actually change the shape of our bones as we strengthen them.

Not only is strength training an essential component to our fitness and flexibility; it is also vital to protect us from the harmful effects of loss of bone density, which can lead to osteopenia and osteoporosis.

Osteopenia is a condition that involves a decrease in bone density. While osteopenia is typically not detrimental to your health, it is considered to be a precursor to osteoporosis. Osteoporosis is a far more serious health threat, because it is a disease that results in significant loss of bone density. Decreased bone density causes thinner, weaker bones that interfere with the mechanical support of the skeleton, particularly the weight-bearing structures of the spine, pelvis, hips, and legs. The bones become extremely vulnerable to fractures and difficult to properly heal when they do break. Not everyone who has osteopenia will develop osteoporosis, but it does place you at higher risk for further bone loss and could be an indication that osteoporosis might be lurking right around the corner. It is not a chance you want to take.

Osteoporosis is most common in postmenopausal women, although it does affect men as well. The effects of osteoporosis can be devastating, with complications that develop as a result of bone fractures, recurring fractures, and surgical procedures required to repair them. Unfortunately, some people do not even realize they have osteoporosis until they have broken a bone. Usually there are no clear visible signs, and osteoporosis can only be diagnosed with a bone density test. However, there is one obvious indicator of osteoporosis, which is a rounding and forward bending of the upper spine between the shoulder blades. This is often referred to as the dreaded "Dowager's Hump," and occurs as a result of the spine collapsing on itself from the weakening structure of the spine. Not only is this extremely painful, it can result in stress fractures of the spine, simply from the act of coughing, sneezing, or even just turning over in bed. The treatment of choice for osteoporosis and osteopenia is medication to prevent further bone loss and rebuild bone strength. However, some of these medications are incredibly expensive, even with insurance coverage, and can have serious undesirable side effects.

Prevention is always worth a pound of cure, and the most reliable and effective method to prevent osteoporosis is to strengthen your bones through weight training. Even if you have already been diagnosed with osteoporosis, you can reverse the process with strength training, as several of my clients have done over the years. However, I will caution you to seek medical advice and appropriate supervision if you have been told you already have a decrease in bone density.

NOTE: Do not try and go it alone; you need help and guidance from a qualified medical professional if you have already been diagnosed with osteopenia or osteoporosis!

Strength training (also referred to as resistance training) comes in many different forms, so I will let you decide for yourself what works best for you. I personally prefer using light weights at home, but you may prefer going to a gym and using the gym's equipment. A lot of gyms and senior centers offer weight training classes for seniors, and many of my clients have gotten terrific results this way.

My most notorious success story came from one of my favorite clients, Clara, who had a long history of osteopenia. One day, when she came in for her weekly Pilates session, she told me she had just received the devastating news that her bone loss had progressed from osteopenia to osteoporosis. Even more discouraging were the nasty side effects she was experiencing from the medication that had been prescribed for her. She asked for my advice, telling me that she didn't know what else she could possibly do to improve her bone health, since she was already doing Pilates once a week and walking every day. I questioned Clara further, asking her if she had been doing the strength training program, using light weights at home, that I had designed for her. No, she admitted. She had other things to do at home and had a difficult time fitting her exercises into her daily routine.

Then I asked her about her walking program, and she assured me that she walked her dog every day. Upon further inquiry, I discovered that walking the dog included stopping for the little guy to sniff every blade of grass that caught his attention. Hmm, not exactly the bone-pounding activity you need to strengthen your bones.

As I kept thinking about options to help Clara, she assured me that she was willing to do absolutely anything to improve her bone health. Finally, I recommended that she take a weight training class for seniors. From the look on her face, it was pretty obvious that she was willing to do anything *but that* and she immediately pooh-poohed the idea. I suppose she underestimated my incomparable stubbornness, because I wouldn't give up on the subject.

Every week I continued to push the idea on her, and every week she rejected it. It took me a few weeks, but eventually she got tired of me nagging her. At long last and with a deeply suspicious look on her face, she agreed to consult with her chiropractor to get her opinion. It was quite apparent that she thought her chiropractor would disagree with me. She was wrong. The chiropractor thought it was a fabulous idea. Crest-fallen and defeated, Clara reluctantly agreed to give it a try.

The first week, she hated it. The second week, she hated it less. By the end of the month, not only was she enjoying it, but she met a lot of new people and was making a lot of interesting new friends as well. Here is the best part of the story: after six months of strength training, her bone density increased and she converted from osteoporosis back to osteopenia and was off her medication. The moral of the story is, "Be careful what you 'pooh-pooh.'"

You have already begun strengthening your body by following the guidelines outlined in the previous five chapters. Once you begin to practice your *Forever Fit and Flexible* program, you will have the correct forces of gravity going through you to help your bones and muscles work collaboratively, all for the power of good. Because of this, you are going to get better results from your strength-training program than you would if you had not built a solid foundation from which to work.

So, in the spirit of trying to keep things simple, as well as effective, I will share some ideas for you to develop a program that you can do at home in just a few minutes a day. You will be surprised at how many opportunities you have during the day to work on strengthening your arms and legs just through performing your functional activities. Once you work with the following strengthening exercises, I encourage you to start experimenting on your own. Look for additional ways to incorporate strengthening exercises into your daily activities.

Remember, strengthening exercises are not just relegated to time in the gym. My paternal grandmother was incredibly strong, and she never saw the inside of a gym. I suppose when you grow up on a farm in Eastern Europe, you learn the meaning and the value of strength through hard work. She continued to do hard physical work every day of her life in her home, yard, and garden. She didn't need a gym, and she probably would have been horrified to think that anyone would need one. If anything, instead of needing a gym, the woman probably needed a rest. However, she retained her strength up until the day she died, and she never did develop osteoporosis.

⌣⌣

The upper body exercises that follow are designed to tone and strengthen your arms, shoulders, upper back muscles, and the muscles between your shoulder blades. This improves your upper body strength as well as your posture and your core muscles. Also, strengthening the area between your shoulder blades takes strain off your neck and shoulders. While we are strengthening and stabilizing our scapular muscles, we need to balance the strength and stability with movement and mobility. Our shoulder blades are meant to slide and glide effortlessly along the back of our rib cage to allow for full range of motion of our neck, head, shoulders, ribs, and spine. This keeps us flexible and supports our posture at the same time. Don't you just love how beautifully this all comes together?

The lower body exercises will help you strengthen and tone the muscles of your buttocks, hips, and legs. Not only will this series of exercises give you strong and shapely legs, it will help you get up and down from sitting with ease and grace. People will wonder what your secret is and what you have been doing to have such youthful vitality. In both the upper body and lower body series, we will add another component of abdominal activation to further strengthen your core. Since we are already working, we might as well get as much benefit as we can from each movement.

Key Points:
- ॐ Strong is sexy.
- ॐ Strong muscles help improve bone strength and increase your metabolism.
- ॐ Strength training can help prevent the devastating effects of osteoporosis.

Checkpoints:
- ॐ Do the exercises slowly and with awareness to achieve the maximum benefit.
- ॐ Focus on proper alignment.

Bonus Points:
- ॐ Practice these exercises intermittently during the day. Just a few repetitions periodically throughout the day really do add up.

FUNCTIONAL STRENGTHENING EXERCISES

This next series of movement lessons are more accurately described as exercises rather than movement lessons. I refer to them as "functional strengthening." They are divided into two sections, one for upper body strengthening and the other for lower body strengthening. The source of these exercises is based on my own personal experiments and my belief that opportunities to strengthen our bodies are everywhere. The only equipment you need for these exercises is a firm chair with armrests. You don't even have to drive to the gym or invest in a set of weights. Not yet, anyway, and not unless you want to.

Movement Lesson #1:
1. **Sit with your sit bones on the edge of a firm chair. Place your feet flat on the floor and your hands on the armrests.**

- Breathe in. As you breathe out, push your hands firmly down on the armrests and begin to straighten your elbows as if you are going to lift yourself up out of the chair. Try not to push with your feet and your legs. Instead, you are trying to do a push-up from a seated position. Hold for a moment, breathe in, and breathe out again as you slowly lower yourself back down into the chair. Take a moment and rest.

- Once again, sit with your sit bones on the edge of the chair, your feet flat on the floor, and your hands on the armrests. Breathe in, and as you breathe out, strongly press your hands down against the armrest in your chair as you push up. In your push-up position, feel your shoulder blades firmly pressing down toward the floor. Hold the position for a moment as you breathe in. Breathe out as you slowly lower yourself back down into the chair. Rest a moment.
NOTE: It is extremely important that your shoulder blades are reaching down toward the floor to stabilize them against your upper back. (This is scapular stability, which was what I assisted the gentleman patient at the nursing home to develop, in order to strengthen the muscles around his shoulder girdle so he could transfer himself and ultimately go home.)

- Again, breathe in. Breathe out as you press your

hands down against the armrest in your push-up. Firmly press your shoulder blades down to the floor at the same time. Keep your arms straight and your shoulder blades pressed down. Keep breathing, hold the position for a slow count of three, and slowly lower yourself down as you breathe out. Stop and rest.

2. **Sit with your sit bones on the edge of a firm chair. Place your feet flat on the floor and your hands on the armrests.**

- Push up from your chair as before and hold the position.

- Keep your arms strong and your elbows straight, but release your shoulder blades and allow your weight to slowly sink down. Then push your hands firmly against the armrests, causing your shoulder blades to press down and your body to lift back up at the same time. You should feel yourself getting taller while you do this. Lower yourself back down on the chair as you breathe out and rest a moment. This will balance your scapular strength and stability with scapular mobility.

- Repeat your push-up and go back and forth from releasing your shoulder blades and sinking your weight down, to pressing hands and shoulder blades down to lift yourself up. Do only a few repetitions, then stop, and lower yourself down to the chair as you breathe out. Stop and rest. You may have already noticed that your lower abdominal muscles are working. Here is a fantastic opportunity to incorporate the strength and awareness of your transverse abdominis that you learned from the chapter on core strength. We will add that component to the exercise.

3. Sit on the edge of your chair with your feet flat on the floor.

- Breathe in, then breathe out and press your hands and shoulder blades down, pulling your lower abdominals in at the same time as you lift yourself up. Firmly engage your lower abdominals as you hold for a slow count of three and then slowly lower yourself back down to your chair.

- Repeat the exercise as above. This time, hold the position for a slow count of five. You can continue to add to your counts, as you feel yourself getting stronger, to further increase your strength and endurance. **NOTE:** Just a few repetitions a day will strengthen, tone, and shape your upper body. As you get even stronger, you can further challenge yourself by lifting your feet off the floor so that your arms are supporting your entire body weight. Who knew that a simple chair provided such incredible opportunities?

Movement Lesson #2:

1. Sit on your chair with your sit bones on the edge of your seat. Place your feet firmly against the floor.

- Without using your arms, slowly shift your weight forward until you feel your feet press even more firmly into the floor. Keep slowly shifting forward until your bottom just barely lifts off the chair; hold it for a moment with your weight balanced over your legs and your legs completely supporting you. Slowly lower yourself back down to the chair. Rest a moment.

- Shift your weight forward until your feet press firmly on the floor. Slowly bring your weight forward over your feet and legs until your bottom barely lifts off the chair. Your knees and hips are bent to support your weight, and your back is straight in the neutral position. Hold for a moment. Slowly lower yourself back down into the chair and rest.

- Shift your weight forward over your feet and legs until your bottom barely lifts off the chair. This time, focus on making the transition of your weight over your feet easy and effortless, rather than lurching yourself forward or using momentum to get there. Hold for a moment and then lower yourself back down to the chair and rest.

- Keeping these points in mind, repeat the exercise. Scoot your weight forward on your chair; slowly lift your weight forward until your bottom just barely lifts off the chair. Hold it for a moment. Slowly lower yourself back down and sit in the chair.

2. Sit on your chair with your sit bones on the edge of your seat. Keep your feet firmly against the floor.

- Slowly shift your weight forward until your bottom lifts slightly off the chair and hold it a bit longer. Make sure that your knees are aligned directly over your toes. In other words, your knees are not rolling in toward each other or out away from each other. Also, make sure that you are bending forward from your hip joints, not rounding your spine. Lower yourself back down to the chair, make yourself comfortable, and rest.

3. Sit on your chair. With your sit bones on the edge of your seat, place your feet firmly against the floor.

~ Slowly shift your weight forward on your chair until your bottom lifts off the chair. Just like you did in the previous exercise, start to engage your transverse abdominis by firmly and gently pulling in your lower abdominals. Keep your neutral spine position. Slowly lower yourself back into the chair.

4. **Sit on your chair. Your sit bones should be on the edge of your seat with your feet firmly against the floor.**

~ Shift your weight forward until your bottom lifts off the chair. Engage your lower abdominals and slowly begin to straighten your knees. Then bend them back to your starting position with your bottom still off the chair. Continue to do slow mini-squats for a count of five to ten repetitions and then lower yourself back into your chair.

Extra Credit:

~ Take a weight training class to further improve your muscle strength and tone. Remember that strong is sexy, at every age.

~ Take a class that teaches the proper way to use light weights at home to further expand your weight training program. Not only is it good for your muscles and your bones, it will enhance your strengthening program. You may be able to find classes through your local community center, parks and recreation center, or senior center. If you cannot find any options that appeal to you or suit your needs, contact a physical therapist in your area to ask them to provide a class as a community service.

chapter eleven

Get Moving and Keep Moving

"Newton knew what he was talking about."

I still have nightmares related to the physics classes I had to take in college. However, Isaac Newton sure knew what he was talking about. He gave us some great advice and insight: "A body in motion tends to stay in motion, while a body at rest …" You get the idea. Once you begin moving, it becomes a habit and a pattern that self-perpetuates. On the other hand, once you stop moving, your metabolism slows down, your muscles atrophy, your joints stiffen up, your breathing is less efficient, and your circulation gets sluggish. Attempting to start to move again feels like trying to start a car that has run out of gas, or a locomotive that has run out of steam.

However, don't get discouraged. It's difficult, but it's not impossible. I do understand that sometimes it is hard to get up and get moving. There were many times in my life when it took monumental effort just to get myself off the couch or out of a chair. Especially if there was a glass of wine or a box of bonbons calling my name. Once I got moving, though, I always felt better physically, mentally, and emotionally.

The point is that you simply have to start moving—and stay moving. Not only is it important for your physical health and well-being, it is essential for your mental and emotional health as well. When you move more, you feel better, you look better, and you think better. The results encourage you to keep moving. A wonderful cycle of positive reinforcement begins, and that is a cycle you want to sustain and nurture.

Walking is a fantastic way to get started on an exercise program. Walking around the park in beautiful weather with a companion can be a rewarding and exhilarating experience. A walk around your neighborhood with your spouse or a neighbor is a great way to spend time with your significant other or a terrific way to bond with your neighbors. A brief walk around the house when the weather is bad is better than not doing anything. Just make the effort to get started. Before you know it, moving will no longer require effort and will become something you find almost effortless to work into your schedule.

If you are not used to physical activity, the key is to start small. If you try to do too much too soon, you can easily become discouraged, overwhelmed, or even injured. Use your awareness to pay attention to how you feel when you exercise. Take note of when it feels right to continue or when your body tells you it is time to stop and take a break. Just as you can do a few repetitions of functional strengthening exercises intermittently during the day, you can incorporate small amounts of physical activity, too. Set small goals that you can commit to and incorporate into your daily activities, and celebrate every accomplishment, no matter how small it may seem to you at the time. Trust me, it really does add up, and it is easy to accomplish.

Here are a few ideas to get you started. When you are running errands or going to the grocery store, park farther away from the storefront. The walk will do you good, and the additional steps quickly begin to accumulate. After dinner, take a brisk walk around your neighborhood before cleaning up the kitchen. When you do clean the kitchen, put on some music and dance around the kitchen as you tidy up. It will make a mundane chore a lot more entertaining and enjoyable. The extra movement has a cumulative effect and will help you get fit.

If you have a sedentary job, make sure you get up and move around the office during the day, as often as possible. Create a schedule for yourself for specific times of the day, such as a mid-morning break, after lunch, etc. You might even set an alarm on your phone or computer to remind you to get up and start moving. Decide what works best for you and make sure that you are consistent with your schedule. Look for opportunities throughout your day to move. For instance, take the stairs instead of the elevator or escalator. After you eat lunch, use your lunch break to take a brisk walk around the building when the weather permits and walk laps around each floor of your office building when the weather is bad. See if your employer will allow you to bring a large exercise ball to work and alternate sitting and gently bouncing on your ball with sitting in your office chair.

One of my clients, Amanda, got the green light from her boss to bring her ball to work because it really helped alleviate her back pain. She had explained to him that it would also help her be more focused and productive, and have less sick days due to back pain. She had a pretty compelling argument, so he'd agreed to allow her to bring her therapy ball to the office. Imagine her astonishment when she came back from lunch earlier than usual one afternoon to find a group of her colleagues playing a lively game of human bowling with her "therapy" ball. Apparently, it was an activity they engaged in whenever she left the office. I asked her if her boss knew what her co-workers were doing with her ball. Amanda replied, "It was his idea." I had to admire their creativity in finding a new use for her ball and a way to get in some exercise, along with some friendly competition at the same time.

Following their example, use your imagination to see how many different and creative ways you can get extra activity in during the day. You might be surprised at what you can come up with, and it may be much more palatable than spending an hour at the gym a few days a week. Besides, if you follow the guidelines in this book, you will experience greater benefits more quickly than if you faithfully go to the gym three times a week. It is not what you do at the gym for those three hours (or more) each week. What really counts is what you do with all those hours in between visits to the gym and how you apply these principles to everyday life.

I like to tell my clients that it is a bit like saving money. Imagine putting a few coins in a piggy bank each and every day. You do not miss it, and it doesn't seem to impact your day-to-day living. However, eventually the coins add up. In time, you find that you have a significant amount of money saved up, yet the process was relatively painless. Compare that to trying to come up with a huge sum of money at one time to put in your savings or to cover an unexpected expense. Getting active and staying active works the same way. Taking small steps on a regular basis is much less painful and far more effective than trying to do large bursts of activity intermittently. Remember, once you start moving, you stay moving. If you stop moving, it takes significantly more effort to start again. Just ask our old friend, Isaac Newton.

The key to continual movement and better health and fitness is to find something you truly enjoy so that you will stick with it. Life is too short to waste time doing something that you hate just because you think it is supposed to be good for you. We are all different. Pursuits that appeal to some of us do not appeal to all of us. Some people seek activities that can be performed in small groups, while others prefer the quiet solitude of individual activities. Still others enjoy being part of a large group or class, or even participating in an organized team sport.

For example, my husband loves organized sports and plays in a competitive men's senior softball league, even though he has two bad knees. It is something he loves to do and has figured out a way to keep playing in spite of his knees.

As I've shared, I personally prefer classes such as dance, martial arts, and Pilates, where I have a lot of social interaction with people who share the same passions as I do. Besides, I need someone to be accountable to, such as an instructor or a workout partner. If I didn't have someone holding my feet to the fire, I would probably sit at home on my couch eating bonbons and wondering why my butt was getting so big and my thighs were turning to mush. Yes, indeed, we all have our issues. So, I am here to encourage you to do what you love, and love what you do. Life is too short to do otherwise. Don't you agree?

Knowing your personal preferences is a great start to sampling a variety of activities that might appeal to you. Narrow your selection down to two or three different activities that you enjoy, and find a way to work them into your schedule. It's really important to choose two or three, instead of just one, because variety is the spice of life, and boredom can kill your enthusiasm for exercise more than anything else will. Besides, a variety of different activities is great cross-training for your body and fantastic cross-training for your brain as well.

If you engage in the same activity over and over, your body becomes used to it and no longer pays attention to what you're doing, because the activity is no longer interesting. Your nervous system does something called "habituation," which simply means that you begin to perform the activity by rote, much like brushing your teeth or washing your face. Because the physical and physiological benefits of the exercise begin to dissipate, you may notice that it becomes repetitive, redundant, and even boring. I recommend doing several activities that have distinct and different movement patterns as a way to challenge and train your body and your brain.

Key Points:
- ❧ Once you start moving, it is easier to stay moving.
- ❧ Adding small amounts of exercise to your daily activities quickly adds up and reaps huge rewards.
- ❧ Celebrate all of your accomplishments, great and small.

Checkpoints:
- ❧ Make sure you are choosing activities that you enjoy and that suit your personality and interests.

Bonus Points:
- ❧ Recruit a friend or two to help keep you on track; you can all support and encourage each other.
- ❧ Remember, it is harder to skip out when you have someone else who is relying on you.

Extra Credit:
- ❧ Enroll in a series of different classes in order to try a variety of activities. You may be surprised by how much fun it can be and how many new friends you make. Besides, I believe you will discover that you love what it does for your body, mind, spirit, and soul.

chapter twelve

Nutrition

"You are what you eat, so keep it
clean, real, fresh, and wholesome."

There is a plethora of information about nutrition swirling
around out there. Unfortunately, most of it is extremely
confusing regarding health, wellness, weight loss, what to
eat, what to avoid, what is going to help you live forever, and
what will probably kill you long before your time.

Often, it is based on the fad of the week combined with
creative advertising that actually undermines our attempts to
eat right and be healthy. There is also a lot of information
about quick and easy weight loss, which often requires you
to buy expensive supplements that promise unbelievable results. The key word is unbelievable, because the only thing
that shrinks is your wallet. There are no magic pills or magic

elixirs for losing weight. However, there is good old-fashioned common sense that will help you the most to achieve your healthy weight. Like everything else, the key to success is awareness and discovering what works best for you. It's also about moderation and finding balance in the process.

Just as an experiment, I encourage you to go to your local bookstore and walk down the nutrition and weight loss aisle. There are so many books available on these subjects that it is mind-boggling. Every author and every method claims to have found the "one and only" right way to weight loss and healthy eating, but incredibly, a lot of them contradict each other. I do not consider myself an expert in the field of nutrition, but I do know how to help you sift through the chaos of information and point you in the right direction. So, allow me to clear things up.

Quite simply, your mom was on the right track when she told you to eat your vegetables, stay away from junk food, and not eat in between meals. She did, however, miss the boat on that last piece of advice. It is much healthier for you to eat smaller meals more often during the day than three large ones. It is easier on your digestion, helps stabilize your blood sugar, and boosts your metabolism. A lot of fit and trim people I know eat small amounts of healthy foods throughout their day. Additionally, they do not deny themselves the pleasure of an occasional treat or even a binge on their favorite food. Once again, life is too short to deny yourself the simple pleasure of eating things that you enjoy. You just want to be aware of what you are eating, and when. The most common mistake that most of us make regarding our eating habits is mindlessly eating when we are not really hungry and making poor choices just because it is convenient or right in front of us.

Here are some ideas to keep in mind as you consider what will work best for you. Be careful not to fall into the trap of following the fads. Do not follow other people's advice, unless they are qualified nutritionists who know what they are talking about, and have your best interests at heart, which includes having a clear understanding of your body and what it needs to function optimally. Instead, listen to yourself. Pay attention to how you feel after you eat certain foods. It is a very important piece of information, and our bodies do have an effective way of communicating with us.

The key is to fine-tune your listening skills so you can hear and process the information you receive. If you feel bloated, sluggish, depressed, or even ill after eating certain foods, they are probably not good for you and best avoided. If you feel satisfied and somewhat energetic, you have likely made good choices that will support your body. Go back to the basics. Stay away from processed foods, and seek out fresh and whole foods. Slowly replace the junk foods with healthier choices. Once again, notice how you feel afterwards. Small, subtle changes are a lot easier to swallow, if you will forgive the expression. They can make a big difference in your overall well-being and will motivate you to take things a few steps further toward a healthier diet.

If weight loss is a primary concern, there are a lot of reputable programs from which to choose. Take time to research them to find the right one for you. You will have better success than going it alone, or buying into the latest sensational weight-loss diet, or adopting a rigid or restrictive diet, such as following a "kale only" diet.

I have nothing against kale, but I do think it's possible to get carried away, which was a lesson I learned a few years ago when I attended a large health fair. I set up my display, which included strategically placing a large basket of dark choco-lates at the front of my table to entice people to come to my booth and talk to me. It wasn't just for the folks attending the event; it was for me as well. After all, it was going to be a long day and I knew I might be in need of some sustenance to keep up my strength. Additionally, there is nothing like the smell of dark chocolate to keep me in a good mood.

I sat down to wait for the event to start and watched the room start to fill up with other vendors. One lady made eye contact with me as she walked by, so I greeted her with a bright smile and a chipper "Good morning!" She responded by looking pointedly at my chocolate and saying in a loud disapproving voice, "Candy … at a health fair! That hardly seems appropriate." She flounced past my booth to set up her table across from me, proudly displaying a variety of fresh produce, including large bunches of kale. Not a bit of choco-late in sight. I guess that explained her reaction to a beautiful basket of chocolates.

Since we were positioned directly across from each other for the entire day, I smiled at her every time she glanced my way. She returned my smile by scowling at my basket of choc-olates, which I had to keep replenishing throughout the day. It was a great event, and I ran out of chocolate long before the day was over. Interestingly, my neighbor never did run out of kale. I felt bad for her, because she didn't seem to be having much fun, and she didn't seem particularly happy. A small piece of chocolate might have even boosted her spirits a bit. The moral of the story is: Do eat your kale, but don't deny yourself a small piece of chocolate every now and then.

It is your personal choice to decide which program is best for you. You can choose from online programs that allow you to customize them to your own personal needs, which may include food selections, exercises, and individual coaching to help you lose weight and get healthy. If you are the type of person who prefers social interaction as well as an opportunity to get away from your computer, check out programs offered in your local community. It is a fabulous way to get help, support, and make a few new friends as well. There is also a lot to be said for having to be accountable to someone. However, make sure that the atmosphere of the group is positive and encouraging. Do you remember the story about my client's weight loss group from earlier in the book? It is no wonder why the group folded. Life is too short to beat yourself up. Besides, it is not healthy. Continual messages that tell you how wrong you are will most likely keep you in self-sabotaging behavioral cycles. They wreak havoc on your self-image, and will surely sabotage your efforts to lose weight.

I remember when my mother began gaining weight many years ago. For a while she tried to ignore it, and then one day she decided to take control again. To get herself back on track, she enrolled in a weight loss class at the local hospital, which she lovingly referred to as her "skinny school." She really liked the fact that, in addition to weight loss, the program focused on providing education regarding nutrition, creating healthy eating patterns, and making good choices. To get into the spirit of being back in school, she recruited her best friend to go with her, so that they could sit together and compare notes, just like they did in high school. They both enjoyed the program and learned a lot of terrific information. Everything was moving along quite well, but after two weeks of classes her friend complained that neither one of them had lost any weight. My mother responded, "Yes, but look at the bright side; neither one of us has gained any in the past two weeks either." Way to stay positive, Mom! Sometimes Mother really does know best.

A picture is worth a thousand words, and I just have to put a plug in for the best weight control book I have ever come across. Notice, I said "weight control" instead of diet, even though the focus of the book is on weight loss. The title of the book is *Picture Perfect Weight Loss* by Dr. Howard M. Shapiro, a physician who specializes in weight control and life management. I keep a copy of his book at home as a reference as well as one at my office to share with my clients.

Dr. Shapiro's approach to weight loss is practical, sensible, positive, easy to follow, and educational. The first thing Dr. Shapiro emphasizes in his program is awareness. Being aware of when you eat, why you eat, and what you eat. As you have already discovered, awareness is the key to success in everything you do, including weight loss and healthy eating habits. In his book, he shows you that you have many choices regarding food selection, and he does it in a way that is without judgment. There is no room for self-incrimination, guilt, or shame—just education and self-awareness. The good doctor even includes strategies for planned binges that you can enjoy without ruining your efforts to stay healthy. Is it any wonder I love this guy? He also includes what he refers to as "secret saboteurs," which are the foods that we think are healthier or lighter in fat or calories, but in fact are the exact opposite. He gives you plenty of food for thought (so to speak), and the opportunity to think again about what you are eating.

The best part of *Picture Perfect Weight Loss* is right there in the title. Through beautiful photographs that really make a long-lasting impression, Dr. Shapiro shows you how to get a lot more food for a lot less calories. One page shows a certain food choice and the calorie count, while the opposite page shows an array of delicious food that equals the same amount of calories, or even less, which you might not even be able to consume at one sitting. The book is a fantastic reference to keep on hand, whether you are trying to lose weight or simply need some new and interesting ideas to perk up your food selection the next time you visit the grocery store. Eating the same things over and over is much like doing the same physical activity over and over again. Your taste buds get bored, and they go into autopilot, making you feel less satisfied and causing you to eat more as a result.

I have another story regarding food that I simply have to share with you. I once worked with two women who worked out together doing Pilates. They were already good friends and spent a lot of time together, so it made sense that they would try and get back into shape together. However, after several weeks of regular Pilates classes, they complained that they were gaining weight and didn't know why. I told them that muscle weighs more than fat, so perhaps that was the reason for the weight gain. Eventually the added muscle tissue would increase their metabolism and help them burn more calories, resulting in a drop in weight. That seemed to make sense to them.

A few weeks later, they reported even more weight gain. Both of them were gaining weight at the same time, and at the same rate. I was confused and quizzed them a bit more about their eating habits. After they assured me that they were both following a healthy diet, they finally admitted that they got together for coffee every afternoon. I was even more perplexed and told them that coffee should not cause them to gain weight, unless they were loading it up with a lot of cream and sugar. (This was long before the advent of triple mocha lattes.) Then they told me the entire story.

Every afternoon they had coffee at a local bakery known for its homemade pies, and pie was an important part of their coffee time. I told them that an occasional slice of pie should not be a problem. It was certainly okay to enjoy a slice of pie every now and then. They then admitted that they didn't have just one piece, but every day they shared an entire pie. Well, that sure did explain the weight gain. I made several different suggestions, including sharing one slice of pie instead of the whole pie, meeting for coffee at a shop that did not offer pie or pastries (good luck with that one), or getting together at each other's home for coffee so there would be no temptation. I also suggested that they meet at a park and go for a walk instead of meet for pie and coffee for their daily girlfriend time.

They dismissed all of my recommendations because they simply had to have the pie, and that was all there was to it. So there! At my wits end, I finally blurted out, "Well then, just quit complaining, eat the pie, and stop feeling guilty about it!" They looked at me like I was crazy. I knew I had just lost two clients, but I couldn't help myself. I took a deep breath and tried again. I said, "Look, you want the pie, you love the pie, and you do not want to give it up. So stop beating yourself up over it. Give yourself permission to eat the pie, and enjoy it. You obviously want the pie more than you want to lose weight. You have made your choice, now be at peace with it."

Not long after my little meltdown, something fascinating happened. I did not lose them as clients. Over the course of the next several months, I noticed that they both began to lose weight. I was almost afraid to ask how they were doing it. When I eventually got up enough nerve to ask them what had changed for them, they told me that they had decided to follow my advice. Once they gave themselves permission to eat as much pie as they wanted and stopped feeling guilty about it, they did not feel compelled to eat it every day. It was no longer forbidden fruit. Even though they still occasionally indulged, it was not the focus of their coffee break. So, I guess you really can have your cake (or pie) and eat it too, as long as you are sensible about it.

Key Points:

- You are what you eat, so keep it real.
- Small changes in your diet are easier to maintain than huge changes.
- It is okay to have an occasional treat, just be sensible about it. Remember to enjoy it when you do, and do not feel guilty about it.

Checkpoints:

- Pay attention to how you feel after you eat certain foods; stick with the ones that energize you, and get rid of the rest.

Bonus Points:

- Take a class on nutrition that includes light and healthy meal planning and preparation.
- Purchase a copy of Dr. Shapiro's book, *Picture Perfect Weight Loss*. It is a great investment.

PART THREE

The Follow-Up Plan

chapter thirteen

Program Review

"When you know what you're doing
you can do what you want."

What follows is an easy reference guide for the *Forever Fit and Flexible* program. Whenever you need a bit of motivation or inspiration, or a quick reminder of any aspect of this program, you can return to this section.

THE FOUNDATION

Awareness

As discussed at the beginning of *Forever Fit and Flexible*, awareness is your key to success in anything and everything you do. Awareness can also help you interrupt habitual patterns that hold you back and open up new possibilities that can help you achieve your goals, whatever they may be.

We all have habits and patterns that we've learned over the years, and some of them are extremely beneficial in helping us get through the day. However, some patterns may not be serving us as well. Consequently, we can change them by bringing our attention to ourselves and realizing when (and how) we may be getting in our own way.

Training your consciousness by becoming more mindful does take some brain power at first, but it gets easier the more you practice it. Once you learn how to be mindful of your patterns, your behavior, and your routine, you can apply a new level of consciousness to all of your physical movements and activities. A surprising and unexpected benefit is how this awareness can then be transferred to other areas of your life. You gain a better understanding of your environment, more clarity in your relationships, and more definition in your goals. It is a life skill well worth developing, and one that will enrich the quality of your life.

Mindset

Our mind and our belief systems have a powerful impact on our physical, mental, emotional, and psychological well-being. Remember that health, wellness, and fitness are measured by how you move and how you feel, rather than a size or a number. Also, remember that life is full of challenges. While we might not be able to change what comes our way, we can certainly change the way we perceive what occurs and how we react. What we believe is what we become, and what we tell ourselves is what we believe. Increase your awareness of everything around you. Pay attention to the messages you send to yourself, or that other people send to you.

You may discover that you are much healthier if you eliminate the negative people in your life. It might be time to let them go so you can grow and thrive. Surround yourself with people who offer positivity to your life and give yourself positive messages too. Celebrate your accomplishments, no matter how small they may seem to you at the time. When you make a mistake, whether it is in your health and fitness program or in any other aspect of your life, please do not beat yourself up. Instead, be kind to yourself! Realize that you are being presented with a wonderful opportunity to learn, so try a different approach. Keep in mind that other people can influence our habits and patterns just as much as what we tell ourselves. Choose your friends well, because negative people can wreak havoc on your self-image and your belief system. Understand that you do not always have to operate from the same habits and patterns as you've operated from in the past, no matter how hard-wired you believe they are. Remember, what you believe is what you become.

Building Your Foundation

Everything starts from the ground up. If you start with a faulty foundation, whatever you put on top of it will make it collapse. The building blocks of a solid foundation include structure, core strength, flexibility, and balance. Together these pillars help to create a solid foundation upon which to move and develop a deeper level of fitness and flexibility.

You create and maintain a solid foundation by starting with neutral alignment of your skeletal structure, also known as correct postural alignment. Remember, healthy posture is easy and effortless, not forced or strained.

The Art of Movement

The movement arts, which have influenced the *Forever Fit and Flexible* program, all share a few common basic principles that make them effective in helping to keep you fit and healthy. Each one of them fully engages your body, mind, and spirit to improve the quality of your movement and the quality of your life.

The benefits, however, go beyond developing physical strength, endurance, balance, flexibility, and energy. These arts also help you gain a greater level of confidence, poise, self-assurance, and resilience. This newfound assurance builds a stronger mental, emotional, and psychological foundation that will help you sustain the heavy loads of life without falling apart. The basic elements presented in *Forever Fit and Flexible* offer you a guide to fitness that is an ongoing process. We are all works in progress, and we are constantly changing. *Forever Fit and Flexible* is a tool to help you build a solid foundation of core strengths that will last a lifetime.

It is important to stay focused and listen to the information your body is communicating to you. These signals will guide you to make adjustments to your program as needed. Remember, this is your opportunity to develop your own program specific to your individual needs and goals. Keep a journal, recording your observations and experiences as you work through each movement lesson. Once you have created your initial program, you have a documented record to refer back to and modify as necessary. Your journal also provides an excellent method to track your progress.

Fundamental Principles

Always keep the basic fundamental principles in mind. I suggest noting them in your journal as a reminder to help you follow them. They will keep you on track, especially if you are running into difficulties, or if you feel like you have reached a plateau in your program. Keep an open mind and approach each challenge with a sense of interest and curiosity. As a quick reminder, here is a summary of the fundamental principles:

1. Each and every movement has a *purpose*.
2. Each and every moment in time deserves its own *attention*.
3. Focus on the *quality* of every movement rather than the quantity or range of motion.
4. Move *slowly*, slower than you have ever moved before.
5. Take frequent *rests*, even though you may feel like you are not doing any work at all and do not need a rest.
6. Allow at least fifteen minutes of uninterrupted time in a *quiet* environment to do each movement lesson.
7. Make yourself *comfortable* as you go through the lessons.
8. Tell yourself you can get there; what we *believe* is what we become.

Remember to listen to yourself instead of following the crowd. If you do, you will stand out and rise above it. Not only does this apply to your quest for fitness and health, but it also has great practical application in many of life's events and situations.

THE PROGRAM

Posture

Posture is the most basic building block of your foundation and your structure. How you stand, move, and walk creates a powerful first impression when you meet new people.

It also communicates to the world how you feel about your-self and what kind of day you are having. More importantly, your posture is essential to your health and wellness as well as your fitness and flexibility. Even if you have struggled with your posture in the past, you can always improve it. It may take some extra thought and determination, but the results will be well worth the effort.

When you stand tall, you look strong, and people take notice. You communicate to the world that you are confident, youthful, and in control. Besides, it makes you feel good!

Core Strength

Strong core muscles help to eliminate and prevent back pain and back injuries. They will strengthen your spine and give you a flatter tummy and smaller waistline. A strong core also helps support your posture and reduces stress and strain on your hips, knees, neck, and shoulders.

You can effectively strengthen your core without the tor-ture of conventional crunches or sit-ups. Core awareness is just as important as core strength, and the ability to isolate and activate your transverse abdominis is the key component to core strength and awareness.

Core strength also refers to your strength of character, your convictions, your personal values, and belief system. Core strength also is a representation of your spirit, which determines who you are as a person, and how you move through life.

Flexibility

Traditional stretching alone will not help you improve your flexibility. You need gentle joint mobilization to lubricate your joints and also to loosen the soft tissue surrounding them. To keep your joints healthy and to keep your muscles functioning with normal tone, you need to use your joints to their fullest range of motion. You can always improve your flexibility simply by getting up and moving around as often as possible during the day. If you do not move it, you will lose it, and it is even more difficult to get it back.

It is also important to exercise your flexibility in how you think and react to life's situations. As Moshe Feldenkrais used to say, "What I am after is not flexible bodies. What I am after is flexible brains."[1] Basically, when you can be flexible in your thinking, you can move through life more easily and effortlessly, even when the going gets rough.

Balance

Balance refers to our ability to adjust quickly and appropriately to changes in our environment, not just the ability to keep ourselves upright. We need to continue to challenge our balance by training the nerve endings in our feet, ankles, hips, and inner ear that respond to our position and our relationship to our environment. Most of us develop a fear of falling as we mature, which can further decrease our balance and equilibrium. Learning how to get down on the floor and back up again can greatly improve your balance as well as your flexibility, and reduce your fear of falling.

Balance goes beyond the physical as well. We have all experienced what it feels like to have the rug pulled out from underneath us, both literally and figuratively. The ability to recover our balance, or to pick ourselves up without getting hurt, is a valuable life skill, no matter what it is that knocked us down.

---

1. Quote from Tubegator Famous Quotes at quotes.tubegator.com

Strength

Strong is sexy, at every age. Forgive me for repeating myself, but I simply cannot help it; I love saying it and I love the sound of it. Not only is a strong body attractive, it exhibits good health and vitality. A strength training program is essential for your health, wellness, and fitness. Strong muscles improve your level of function and increase your energy, endurance, and metabolism. Fit, healthy muscles are resilient and help prevent injuries as well as bone loss and the devastating effects of osteoporosis.

You are going to get even better results from strength training as a result of improving your posture, core strength, flexibility, and balance. Now that the forces of gravity are going through you in a more efficient manner, your muscles and bones are already improving in strength and endurance. It's time to further shape and tone your muscles with resistance training in the form of using light weights at home, joining a weight training class for seniors, or using the equipment at a gym if that's your preference. Also, remember to look for opportunities to add resistance training into your schedule and daily activities, because opportunities are everywhere. When you consider the alternatives, there really is no excuse not to do so.

Strength, as well, goes beyond the physical. Strength is more than having strapping muscles and a fit body. It includes having a powerful mind, a resilient spirit, and a staunch belief system of who you are, what you need, and how to get it.

Get Moving and Stay Moving

You just cannot fight the laws of physics. They are working for you, not against you. Remember that a body in motion tends to stay in motion, and once you get started, you will not even want to stop. Choose a variety of different activities to challenge yourself and keep your body and your brain from getting bored. Remember to explore activities that suit your interests and personality. Recruit a friend to try some classes with you at your recreational center or adult learning center. Or, go it alone and find an entirely new group of friends that share your same interests and passions. You never know who you might meet.

Movement is life, and life is a process. Make every move count, and look for every opportunity to keep moving. It will keep you fit and healthy in body, mind, and spirit.

Nutrition

Remember, you are what you eat, so you want to stick to foods that are real, fresh, and wholesome. Stay away from the junk food, since it will wreak havoc on your physical health and ruin your cognitive and mental health as well. Pay attention to how you feel after eating unwholesome foods, and eliminate them from your diet. Make small, gradual changes if you need to, rather than radically changing your diet all at once. Small changes have more staying power and will help you get used to your new changes. Stay away from the fads. Instead of following the crowd, follow what makes sense to you, and what feels right for you. If you need to lose weight, do your research and find out what is available in your community. Remember, you will have greater success if you keep it positive.

Good nutrition goes beyond food. Just as you are what you put into your body, you are what you put into your mind. Take the time to nourish your brain and mind, just as you nourish your body.

chapter fourteen

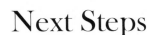

Next Steps

"Are we there yet?"

When I was growing up, a family vacation meant packing up the car and taking a long road trip to our destination. Everyone we knew traveled that way, since air travel was considered quite extravagant, especially when adding up airfare for a family of five or more. Besides, most of the places we went for vacations or family visits could be reached in just a few hours by car.

Unfortunately, to a child crammed between siblings and suitcases in a car with no air conditioning, a few hours seemed interminable. No matter where we were going, my parents were subjected to the recurrent and plaintive whine from the back seat, "Are we there yet?" Since my siblings and I grew up in a generation without a variety of technology and videos to distract us, our parents had to try different strategies to keep us quiet. It was no different for the families of friends and relatives of those times.

I remember one summer when my three cousins were getting ready to take off for their annual summer vacation. Before they got in the car, my uncle lined them up on their front porch and gave them a stern lecture about where they were going and exactly how long it would take to get there. He finished his admonition with the warning that under no circumstances did he want to hear the words, "Are we there yet?" He even threatened to turn the car around and head straight back home if any of them even whispered the forbidden words. They hadn't even made it outside the city limits of our small town before my youngest cousin uttered the dreaded phrase in her most solemn voice, "Are we there yet?"

When my family took a road trip, my mother invented car games to keep us entertained. She was incredibly creative, but my sisters and I still got bored pretty quickly. Besides, playing car games with our siblings, when we were already sick of each other, just made being immobilized in a car, with a long stretch of highway ahead, even more unbearable. All we could think was, "Are we there yet?" However, unlike my young cousin, we knew better than to ask. Instead, we sat and squirmed, and tried to pick at and bug each other as quietly as possible.

During one particularly long trip, my sisters and I were rolling around in the back of the family station wagon. Of course, this was long before mandatory seat belt laws and child seats. One of my sisters decided that we should line up and sit like we were sitting in our seats, but face backward. We got a lot of attention from the passengers in other vehicles, just as my sister had hoped. However, what had started as a joke turned out to be an incredibly eye-opening experience.

We were fascinated by looking at where we had been rather than where we were going. We were far more interested in the miles we had put behind us as we focused on the scenery speeding past us rather than the long stretch of road ahead. We became just as interested in the journey as the destination, and our parents never again heard that petulant query, "Are we there yet?" From that moment on, anytime we became restless during a road trip, we turned ourselves around so we could appreciate how far we had come.

It's hard to be patient when you are excited to get to where you're going, but focusing on the journey, as well as the progress you make along the way, makes the process more interesting and rewarding. The journey to being *fit and flexible* is a lot like those car trips. We are so anxious to get to the end result that we forget to remember how far we've come.

Now is the time to reflect upon where you were when you started this journey. Look back on where you have been and what you have done. Read back over your journal and review your notes. Reflect on the progress you've made as well as the obstacles you've encountered along the way. Notice what you've done for yourself or how you may have modified the movement lessons or your approach to the lessons to make this program uniquely yours. Keep looking back even as you move forward to evaluate your program.

And just as you would when planning a trip, look ahead to where you're going from here. Add new challenges as you make progress to avoid mindlessly going through your program or getting bored. When we are striving toward the goal to be *forever fit and flexible* we never really get to the end.

With that in mind, consider where you would like to be as you move forward. Where are you going in the future and what would you like that to look like? Write down your goals, dreams, and aspirations. Come up with ideas for how you can achieve them. Keep in mind that you can do anything you put your mind to, and don't let anyone tell you that you can't.

The journey to being *Forever Fit and Flexible* is a continuous one, and one that requires our constant attention. However, this journey can be surprisingly easy as well as fun, as long as we approach it with a sense of interest, inquisitiveness, and self-education. Fitness and flexibility are more than a size or a number. They represent a frame of mind, a way of life, and a belief system. We are all getting older, but we do not have to get old. I envision an entire society of men and women over fifty who are able to enjoy a quality of life and a level of activity that they might never have dreamed possible.

Once you make the commitment to be *fit and flexible*, there is no limit to what you can do for yourself. You now have the tools to help you find your way and to discover what works best for you. It is my firm belief that anyone can be fit, flexible, healthy, vibrant, and energetic. With each new decade of life that you celebrate, whether your fifties, sixties, seventies, or beyond, tell yourself that the best is still yet to come. Enjoy the journey!

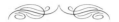

Acknowledgments

I am forever grateful to the many people who have shaped my life and influenced me in my journey to fitness and flexibility, especially those who have supported me in the idea for this book.

To my husband, Mike, who has stood by my side through the good times, the bad times, and the really crazy times. Thank you for being my husband, my partner, my advisor, and my friend. I love you!

To my sister Alyssa, who has said time and time again, "You should write a book someday." Thank you for your support, for your faith in me, and for always having my back. You are amazing!

To my niece Taylor and my nephew Dylan, who inspire me to keep *fit and flexible* so I can keep up with you. Thank you for being the best playmates I've ever had! Your Aunt Cheryl adores you.

To my Aunt Stella, who has always been a fantastic role model and a great example. You taught me that not only is it possible to balance work, family, and bowling, but you can do it with grace and style. We all want to be Aunt Stella when we grow up.

Finally, to all my wonderful clients who have given me the honor and privilege of working with you over the years. Thank you for coming into my life and into my heart. I am grateful to each and every one of you.

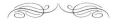

About the Author

Cheryl Ilov has always been drawn to health and wellness, the biological sciences, and movement arts, including classical ballet. She began her professional life as a respiratory therapist, and after seventeen years of practice, she returned to school and earned her master's degree in physical therapy in 1996.

Cheryl discovered The Pilates Method in 1983, and once she began working as a physical therapist, she made the connection that Pilates presented a wonderful tool to help people of all ages recover from injuries and illnesses. She immediately began applying the principles of Pilates to her patients to improve their quality of life and level of function. In 1999, she founded Ilov Integrated Arts, specializing in Pilates-based rehabilitation.

Cheryl had her first experience with The Feldenkrais Method® in 2000. She began the required four-year training program to become a Feldenkrais practitioner in February 2006 and graduated in November 2009. During Cheryl's remarkable journey of learning, healing, and self-discovery, she also discovered a martial art called Ninpo Tai Jutsu. She fell in love with the art and the training as well as the powerful connection between Feldenkrais and martial arts and their incredible healing power.